Studies in Computational Intelligence

Volume 909

Series Editor

Janusz Kacprzyk, Polish Academy of Sciences, Warsaw, Poland

The series "Studies in Computational Intelligence" (SCI) publishes new developments and advances in the various areas of computational intelligence—quickly and with a high quality. The intent is to cover the theory, applications, and design methods of computational intelligence, as embedded in the fields of engineering, computer science, physics and life sciences, as well as the methodologies behind them. The series contains monographs, lecture notes and edited volumes in computational intelligence spanning the areas of neural networks, connectionist systems, genetic algorithms, evolutionary computation, artificial intelligence, cellular automata, self-organizing systems, soft computing, fuzzy systems, and hybrid intelligent systems. Of particular value to both the contributors and the readership are the short publication timeframe and the world-wide distribution, which enable both wide and rapid dissemination of research output.

The books of this series are submitted to indexing to Web of Science, EI-Compendex, DBLP, SCOPUS, Google Scholar and Springerlink.

More information about this series at http://www.springer.com/series/7092

Utku Kose · Omer Deperlioglu ·
Jafar Alzubi · Bogdan Patrut

Deep Learning for Medical
Decision Support Systems

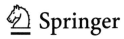 Springer

Utku Kose
Department of Computer Engineering
Süleyman Demirel University
Isparta, Turkey

Omer Deperlioglu
Department of Computer Technologies
Afyon Kocatepe University
Afyonkarahisar, Turkey

Jafar Alzubi
Faculty of Engineering
Al-Balqa Applied University
Al-Salt, Jordan

Bogdan Patrut
Faculty of Computer Science
Alexandru Ioan Cuza University of Iasi
Iasi, Romania

ISSN 1860-949X   ISSN 1860-9503 (electronic)
Studies in Computational Intelligence
ISBN 978-981-15-6327-0   ISBN 978-981-15-6325-6 (eBook)
https://doi.org/10.1007/978-981-15-6325-6

This Springer imprint is published by the registered company Springer Nature Singapore Pte Ltd.
The registered company address is: 152 Beach Road, #21-01/04 Gateway East, Singapore 189721, Singapore

Foreword by Dr. Deepak Gupta

Artificial intelligence is briefly an engineering perspective for designing and developing flexible and robust solutions, which can be widely applied to real-world-related problems. As associated with many remarkable technologies such as computer, communication, and electronics, outputs of the field of artificial intelligence has already been seen in different areas at the start of the twenty-first century. Now, it can be seen that the use of artificial intelligence is in its way to be a common thing used widely by people during daily life. That is because innovative devices gained great rise as a result of more increases in need for using, changing and changing the information even instantly worldwide. By the way, effective advantages of artificial intelligence-based methods and techniques for automated decision-making have been taking researchers' interests for a very long time, as taking us back to even starting times of the artificial intelligence. It seems that the decision support will be one of the most critical roles of artificial intelligence-based systems of the future because more intense digital data requires automated analysis and evaluation phases as it may take time and be very difficult for humans to make that even without errors. Because of that we can see active uses of decision support systems in both natural and social sciences, and the field of medical is among them as it includes decision-making phases during symptom analyzes, diagnosis, and treatment.

It is a pleasure for me to write a foreword for this book as it includes recent achievements and skills–knowledge combination in the context of deep learning and medical decision support systems. As the current, more advanced form of the machine learning, the deep learning is a wide collection of neural networks currently, and it is applied with improved success rates in problems of medical. Thanks to its relation with especially data processing techniques; it has been even easier and faster to get better, more accurate and effective outcomes for the medical applications. In that context, this book takes readers from brief introduction to the essential concepts, and then goes with diagnosis-related different applications including uses of different deep learning techniques as well as different diseases in the target. It is good to see that all subjects covered in the book are explained in enough technical details and giving further information about what can be learned and how to proceed next. The chapters also generally get combinations of deep learning and data processing to ensure automated diagnosis so that medical decision supports accordingly. I suggest the readers to have a start from Chap. 1, and then read the Chaps. 2–9 for better learning about skills for performing alternative research. I liked also that the final Chap. 10 have a final discussion about future perspectives for the future of medical decision support systems and also give a scenario for using current and future technologies for tracking and controlling pandemics, as it is very critical because the world and the existence of the human is nowadays under the attack by the COVID-19, which is a fatal virus type.

I suggest the book to be used during the courses regarding the fields of computer science/engineering, medical and biomedical engineering, and also it will be a good reference for the data science-oriented courses, too. The level of technical details and the used language is all appropriate for the students at the level of B.Sc., M.Sc., Ph.D., and also post-docs. I take interests the readers to also suggestions made by the authors at the end of each chapter, in order to continue improving their knowledge.

I would like to thank Dr. Utku Kose and his co-authors Dr. Omer Deperlioglu, Dr. Jafar Alzubi, and Dr. Bogdan Patrut for their valuable work and also wish the readers to have enjoyable learning as well as research experiences with the support of that book.

Dr. Deepak Gupta
Maharaja Agrasen Institute of Technology
New Delhi, India
e-mail: deepakgupta@mait.ac.in

Foreword by Dr. Jose Antonio Marmolejo-Saucedo and Dr. Igor Litvinchev

Recent advances in information technologies result in evolution of decision support systems involving various techniques for analyses and handling big data. These systems are applied in a broad range of disciplines, e.g., in administration, engineering, and health systems.

In the field of medical informatics, designing and developing tools to support decision-making were highly motivated by advances in biometrics. Among different applications in health systems, medical diagnostics is especially important. Diagnostics is often challenging since many signs and symptoms are hidden and nonspecific. To cope with this problem, a correlation of the information must be analyzed, combined with recognition and differentiation of patterns. Algorithms for data analysis are among various techniques used in diagnostic procedures. Among them, neural networks and deep learning approaches play an important role. In medical diagnostics, the deep learning frequently provides more robust results comparing with the artificial neural networks. The deep learning techniques were successfully used for cancer diagnostics. Many other fields of medicine are also open for high-level decision support systems that can diagnose and treat better than humans.

In this book, different medical data handling techniques are used to develop medical decision support systems in the context of diagnosis perspective. The objective is to use all available information in the decision-making to improve the quality of medical care and to help less experienced doctors in diagnostics.

Challenges and problems associated with implementations of medical decision support systems are discussed, as well as strategies for their development and validation. The book describes theoretical foundations used for developing decision support systems. Basic information on medical diagnostics in different situations is also presented. Finally, perspectives of medical decision support systems are discussed and related with that of the progress in artificial intelligence, deep learning, and modern innovative technologies such as Internet of Health Things.

Today, epidemics like COVID-19 have tested the ability of health systems to meet the new challenges. This book provides a valuable impact in the developing medical decision support systems and with this in obtaining better solutions for the future.

Dr. Jose Antonio Marmolejo-Saucedo
Universidad Panamericana
Mexico City, Mexico
e-mail: jmarmolejo@up.edu.mx

Dr. Igor Litvinchev
Nuevo Leon State University
San Nicolás de los Garza, Mexico
e-mail: igor.litvinchev@uanl.edu.mx

Preface

Deep learning is currently the biggest problem solution way and the technology side of the field of artificial intelligence. As a result of increased uses of digital world and the digital data created with the tasks done in that world, it has been a great necessity to run more advanced form of machine learning. Thus, the concept of deep learning has been designed in order to define advanced forms of neural networks, which is the most successful technique of machine learning. Maybe, the future will bring us different techniques of deep learning, as out of the neural network modeling approach, but it is clear that the deep learning has a remarkable popularity nowadays, and it seems that it will be still widely applied in competitive problems in the future.

There are many different fields where artificial intelligence and the deep learning are intensively used. Main purposes of uses are generally related to improvements/increases in terms of successful outcomes, effectiveness, efficiency, and further technological developments. As in the context of these purposes, the field of medical is one of the most critical fields where artificial intelligence and deep learning are used. From pre-analyses of medical data to diagnosis, from diagnosis to the whole treatment phases, it is possible to see wide employments of intelligent systems in order to reach to the desired results at the end. As we have already given emphasis to the deep learning, it can be clearly said that deep learning techniques—architectures are effectively used nowadays for dealing with medical problems. By gathering all of the applications in one hand, we can also indicate that the decision support approach has the highest priority in the context of performed research works.

By combining deep learning and medical decision support systems together, we introduce our book study: Deep Learning for Medical Decision Support Systems, to the readers' valuable consideration. We have combined essentials of the main topics, direct explanations for the uses of deep learning solutions in the view of diagnosis, and eventually tried our best to get a good reference book, which can be used by scientist, experts, students in different degrees, and of course anyone interested to get informed about the covered topics and the most recent state of the associated literature in terms of medical diagnosis processes to ensure the medical support.

We can explain briefly the covered topics in each of the next chapters as follows:

Chapter 1 makes a fresh start to the book by explaining some about artificial intelligence and its role in development of decision support systems. The chapter finalizes its discussion by making connection to the deep learning.

Chapter 2 gives a deep explanation regarding essentials of the widely used deep learning architectures such as convolutional neural network (CNN), recurrent neural network (RNN), autoencoder network (AEN), deep neural network (DNN), and the deep belief network (DBF) as used in the context of medical diagnosis.

Chapter 3 takes the explanations in the previous chapter one-step away and focuses on some recent and remarkable applications of the deep learning architectures–methods used in medical diagnostics for common areas.

Chapter 4 explains a diagnosis approach for the diabetic retinopathy with a deep learning method by using image processing over the colorful retinal fundus images from the Messidor Database and also apply of the convolutional neural network (CNN).

Chapter 5 investigates the diagnosis of Parkinson's disease with a deep learning approach by using the data obtained from the dataset of the Oxford Parkinson Diagnosis, as in the form of sound data.

Chapter 6 focuses on the detection of heart diseases using the Cleveland Heart Disease data set and use of the autoencoder network (AEN) for diagnosis so that it can be shown that the classification success can be increased easily by using AEN without any feature selection process or mixed methods.

Chapter 7 introduces a hybrid system for medical diagnosis. In this sense, a swarm intelligence supported autoencoder-based recurrent neural network (ARNN) has been explained for ensuring a flexible multi-diagnosis system called as SIARNN briefly.

Chapter 8 explains a use of long short-term memory (LSTM) model and facial expression detection approach for ensuring a psychological personal support system, which can perform some analyzes with question–answer period or image-viewing sessions, to get some idea about emotional changes shown by the target person.

Chapter 9 revisits the diagnosis of diabetic retinopathy, and that time, it explains the use of image processing and the Capsule Network (CapsNet), which is a recent deep learning technique, for ensuring effective diagnosis at the end.

Chapter 10 concludes the book by analyzing future perspective of the medical decision support systems by evaluating progress of artificial intelligence, deep learning, and discussing about future components such as Internet of Health Things (IoHT), wearable technologies, robotics, drug discovery, rare disease/cancer diagnosis. The chapter also gives a future scenario perspective against the current world-wide problem: COVID-19 virus and pandemic control in general (We hope that will be a helpful contribution for fighting against the COVID-19).

Now we invite all readers to turn the pages for getting a wide, recent view on the world of deep learning and its applications on diagnosis-related works to achieve medical decision support eventually. Ideas and valuable feedback from readers are always welcome, and we hope you will all like reading the next chapters. We also would like to thank to Profs. Gupta, Marmolejo-Saucedo, and Litvinchev for their kind and valuable forewords.

Authors

Isparta, Turkey

Dr. Utku Kose

utkukose@sdu.edu.tr

http://www.utkukose.com

Afyonkarahisar, Turkey

Dr. Omer Deperlioglu

deperlioglu@aku.edu.tr

Al-Salt, Jordan

Dr. Jafar Alzubi

j.zubi@bau.edu.jo

Iasi, Romania

Bogdan Patrut

bogdan@info.uaic.ro

bogdan@edusoft.ro

Acknowledgements As the authors, we would like to thank Loyola D'Silva, Swetha Divakar, and the Springer Team for their valuable efforts and great support on pre-organizing the content and publishing of the book.

About This Book

Artificial intelligence is currently used within all fields of the modern life, and especially machine learning has a great popularity since it includes techniques that are capable of learning from samples to solve newly encountered cases. Nowadays, a recent form of machine learning: deep learning is widely used over complex, higher amount of data because today's problems require detailed analyses of more data. That is critical for especially fields such as medical. Moving from that, objective of this authored book is to provide essentials and some recent uses about deep learning architectures for medical decision support systems. The book consists of a total of 10 chapters providing recent knowledge regarding introduction to the main topics of the book, different applications of deep learning-oriented diagnosis leading to decision support, and some ideas regarding the future state of the medical decision support systems. The target audience of the book includes scientists, experts, M.Sc. and Ph.D. students, post-docs, and any readers interested in the covered subjects. The book is appropriate to be used as a reference work during the courses of artificial intelligence, machine/deep learning, medical as well as the biomedical.

Utku Kose
Omer Deperlioglu
Jafar Alzubi
Bogdan Patrut
(Authors)

Contents

Chapter 1
Artificial Intelligence and Decision Support Systems

The humankind has always found its way on solving problems in the real-world, by using tools and deriving solution scenarios. As the more tools designed and developed by humans, the more effective solutions and new kinds of tools for better solutions were obtained always. Eventually, the humankind started to use the concept of technology for defining all kinds of knowledge and skills employed for designing as well developing solutions for different fields [1, 2]. It is critical that the humankind started to give meaning to the life by examining it under different fields and the technologies used for making problem solutions and experiences within these fields easier—more practical. It is also important that the following features and mechanisms of the technology has been important on historical rise of the life standards [3–6]:

- Technology is a dynamic concept adapting itself to the changed conditions,
- Technology has not any direct—specific field scope (it may affect everything in a vertical and horizontal way),
- Each technology has the ability to affect every different technology,
- Technology has both theoretical aspects (knowledge) and applied aspects (skills) to make the life better,
- Technology is a universal concept.

Considering the mentioned features and mechanisms, Fig. 1.1 provides a general view of the characteristics of the technology.

Based on the explanations so far, it is possible to indicate that the humankind is currently surrounded by many different technologies. These technologies are generally somehow ensuring different levels of focus in the context of fields of the modern life. As associated with the current technological state of the twenty-first century, it can be expressed that both computer and communication technologies had had revolutionary changes in technological manner. As related to computers and even supportive components such as electronics, modern logic, mathematics on the background, the field of Computer Science has a long-time rise to shape the currently experienced technological state.

© The Editor(s) (if applicable) and The Author(s), under exclusive license to Springer Nature Singapore Pte Ltd. 2021
U. Kose et al., *Deep Learning for Medical Decision Support Systems*,
Studies in Computational Intelligence 909,
https://doi.org/10.1007/978-981-15-6325-6_1

Fig. 1.1 Characteristics of
the technology

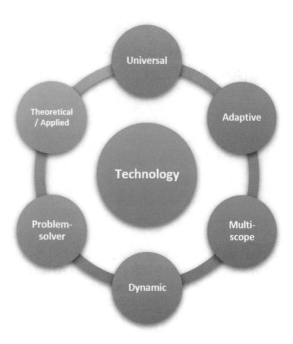

In the context of the Computer Science, there are different sub-fields where different theoretical and applied aspects of the Computer Science are widely discussed. As the computer technology has a triggering role in technological developments for a very long time, the role of Computer Science is important as a main research target for the scientific audience. As including the engineering aspects, Computer Science and Engineering has been an effective ground for the effective tools, and devices people using to deal with the real world, by using also power of the digital world.

Among all sub-fields of the Computer Science, artificial intelligence has a top place since it has many advantages to ensure successful applications for all fields of the modern life. As one of the most vital fields associated with the human life and the nature, the field of medical here has a strong relation with artificial intelligence. There are many different application types that can be associated with common use of artificial intelligence and medical but all these applications lead to the decision support making as humans still has the control (widely or narrowly depending on the target medical problems) at the end. As the first chapter of the book, a fresh start will be done in the context of this chapter, by providing brief explanations regarding artificial intelligence and its sub-research areas as machine/deep learning, and the role of intelligent systems in developing decision support systems, which are used within also medical.

1.1 Artificial Intelligence and Intelligent Systems

With a brief and direct definition, Artificial intelligence can be defined as the field of designing and developing systems, that can provide effective solutions for real world problems, by inspiring from human thinking—behaviors as well as actions by other living organisms and dynamics observed in the nature [7–9]. Artificial intelligence is a product by the humankind as it is very effective and efficient tools for getting automated solutions for real-world problems. As the humankind have many discoveries and inventions in the past, the artificial intelligence is the latest revolutionary invention gave a great rise to the technological developments started from middle of the twentieth century. Considering the current state of the twenty-first century, there is not any fields where artificial intelligence-based approaches, methods, and techniques are not used. In the form of just iterative code groups, it has been like a very easy task to solve difficult (and even almost impossible) problems, by employment of artificial intelligence. All these are because of some important characteristics (like the technology have as shown in Fig. 1.1) of the artificial intelligence. Figure 1.2 briefly expresses these characteristics.

Characteristics of the artificial intelligence has made that field effectively used tool for different fields where problems can be modeled mathematically and logically as the life itself is a typical chaos that has the meanings in terms of mathematics and the modern logic. In detail, the solution ways provided by artificial intelligence follows the chance factor as a heuristic view on getting solutions. These solutions are

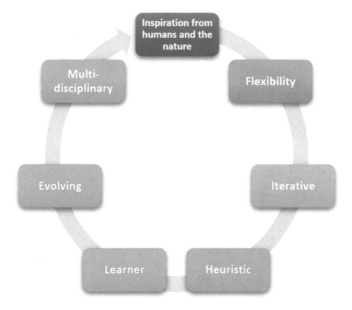

Fig. 1.2 Essential characteristics of the artificial intelligence

done in an iterative manner, by using learning steps causing an artificial intelligence-based technique-system to get enough idea about how to solve the target problem, and learn about the latest changes about the problem so that improving experience in an evolving manner. By taking the support of mathematically and logically structured algorithmic steps, all these allows multi-disciplinary applications as a result of flexibility.

Artificial intelligence is strong enough because it also has great relation with alternative fields and technologies. Solutions in the context of artificial intelligence often needs tasks to be done over target data (of the problem) so that there have been a remarkable relation with data processing approaches (image processing/signal processing), and at the end the outcomes of the artificial intelligence have become useful for introduce of different fields—technologies or sub-areas such as data mining, cybernetics, and robotics. Figure 1.3 represents a general view of that relation and the world of the artificial intelligence as generally. That view can be improved by including more relations as the artificial intelligence has a great—good relation in the context of its surroundings.

Currently, artificial intelligence is a typical mixture of different solution approaches, methods under these approaches, and also techniques—algorithms based on different methods. Except from detailed roots, it is possible to indicate that an artificial intelligence-based system can achieve the followings in the time of solving real-world problems [10–14]:

- Pattern recognition,
- Prediction/estimation,

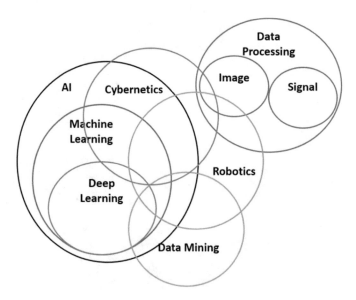

Fig. 1.3 Artificial intelligence and its relations

- Data discovery,
- Data transformation,
- Optimization,
- Adaptive control,
- Diagnosis.

All these problem solution ways are essential for artificial intelligence generally. But on the other hand, diversities among different techniques—algorithms and the followed methods have caused some sub-areas to be introduced under the field of artificial intelligence.

1.1.1 Areas of Artificial Intelligence

Although there are many detailed perspectives to explain sub-areas of artificial intelligence, an easier explanation can also be done accordingly. In this sense, artificial intelligence techniques are generally divided into two categories first: (1) learning techniques, (2) direct techniques. The learning techniques caused the machine learning sub-area to rise, as the most important solution approach of the artificial intelligence. In many problem solutions, the concept of machine learning is directly used for expressing the active use of artificial intelligence. Machine learning is also currently still rising with the advanced forms of techniques under deep learning [15–20]. On the other hand, direct techniques of artificial intelligence include general techniques such as fuzzy logic or natural language processing techniques and there is also intelligent optimization as the optimization-oriented solutions by the artificial intelligence [21–23]. Figure 1.4 provides a general scheme regarding to that classification/sub-areas of the artificial intelligence.

1.1.2 Intelligent Systems

The concept of intelligent system may be used for defining logically a whole artificial intelligence-based system, by eliminating technical details such as which processes and algorithms are run in the system. As artificial intelligence is now at the edge of being a common thing in daily life, such general concepts are fine to be used for indicating active use of artificial intelligence-based solutions in different domains. An intelligent system can be in the form of only software or hardware supported with the software infrastructure. Intelligent system can be a problem-specific use of a certain technique or a hybrid formation with use of more than one artificial intelligence technique or combinations of both artificial intelligence techniques and alternative solutions from different fields. Turning back to the logical meaning of intelligent systems, these systems allows people to receive interactions regarding

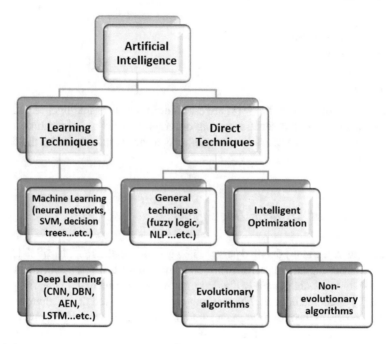

Fig. 1.4 Areas/sub-areas of artificial intelligence

Fig. 1.5 Solution ways by
intelligent systems

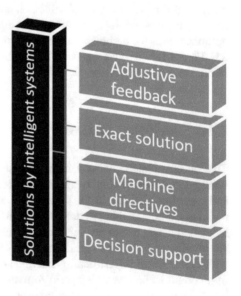

some kind of solution ways. Figure 1.5 represents a general list of these solution
ways.

Moving from Fig. 1.5, it can be said that an intelligent system can provide some adjustive values/solutions for an instant run of another system or making that system—component better at the end. On the other hand, the intelligent system can make it work by providing a final solution to be used independently. Also, it is possible for an intelligent system to get some machine—device-oriented directives to control other electronic/electro-mechanic systems as it is seen as an interaction among machines—devices from the human view. Finally, an intelligent system can provide decision support, which means the provided solutions can be used to get a final decision or finalize a diagnosis.

1.2   Decision Support Systems

Decision making has always been a problem for people. At the time of especially critical decision making, it is important to eliminate different factors such as stress, noise, illness, or fatigue, in order to get an accurate and true decision at the end. In even decisions made in appropriate cases, different environmental factors may cause unpredicted results later. So, the subject of decision making has always been a critical topic for the research works [24–26]. At this point, the technology use has also brought many advantages to make decision making processes faster and easier, thanks to use of computer technologies and data analyzing—processing approaches. As appropriate to that, decision support systems have been developing in order to support people in different fields, for making automated decisions or at least using an assistive software system for getting advices. As general, a decision support system (DSS) can be defined as a system, which can automatically process and analyze some input data in order to reach to a decision as the output [27–29]. Because artificial intelligence is highly associated with ensuring effective and accurate DSS, such systems have been providing as in the form of intelligent systems. Figure 1.6 provides an example of a structure for a DSS [30].

Because decision making is done generally in all fields, the literature has many alternative DSS models and research works done so far. Some of remarkable fields where DSS are widely used can be listed as follows:

- Finance [31–34],
- Business Management [35–39],
- Energy [40–44],
- Education [45–47],
- Environmental Engineering [48–50],
- Medical [51–57].

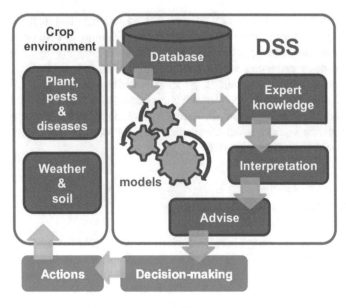

Fig. 1.6 An example of decision support system [30]

1.2.1 Decision Support Systems for Medical and Deep Learning

Recently, there is a great need for running DSS for ensuring effective solutions for medical problems. As it was expressed before, use of artificial intelligence in the context of daily life can be meaningful for non-expert people by using logical concepts. As similar, the concept of DSS is widely used in medical applications and researched widely by the scientific audience. It is clear that the current and future state of medical with artificial intelligence includes remarkable use of DSS solutions [58–60]. As general, DSS can be used in the context of medical by focusing the related factors shown in Fig. 1.7 [58–62].

As explained under the previous paragraphs, there are typical formations of DSS but in terms of medical, it is critical to meet with the listed factors. After designing the exact infrastructure of intelligent system in the context of software approach, it is easier to add frontend. Because of that, this book gave more emphasis to the solutions itself. Also, the systems explained under the next sections of the book are generally focused on disease diagnosis factor, as the processes leading to the diagnostics already employs the other factors of data-oriented works and the personal support (in terms of doctors, medical staff, and the patient) already.

Because DSS has high relations with artificial intelligence, developments in the field of artificial intelligence directly affects the way of DSS research. As a DSS requires evaluation of known samples or learning from the obtained data for having a decision finally, machine learning related methods and techniques are widely used in

Fig. 1.7 Using factors of decision support systems in medical

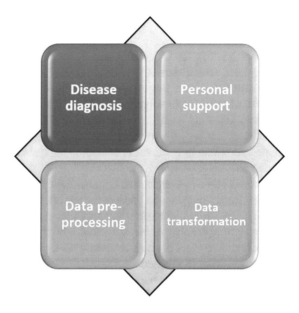

the context of DSS. As similar, the latest form of machine learning: deep learning has been intensively employed for designing and developing innovative DSS approaches and supporting the field of medical in this way [63–65]. The advantages of deep learning within DSS are associated with the advantages by deep learning techniques. Figure 1.8 represents these advantages generally.

Fig. 1.8 Advantages of deep learning in medical decision support systems

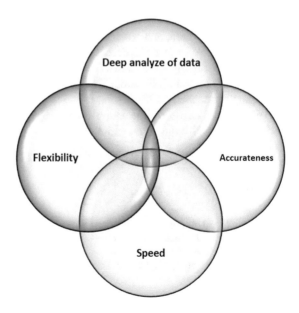

1.3 Summary

Artificial intelligence is a top field shaped the technological developments. As it is associated with different application types rising over different problem solution perspectives, it seems to be used more and more in the near future. Additionally, the field of artificial intelligence has already strong sub-areas as machine learning and deep learning. Thanks to the learning capabilities of machine/deep learning techniques, it is possible to solve even advanced problems and developing effective enough solutions in the context of intelligent systems, as a logical concept known by people.

This chapter made an introduction to the essentials of artificial intelligence (as within wide-narrow enough borders for this book) and then explained the concept of decision support systems with their application fields as including also medical. As the final touch, the chapter has also made a brief open for the use of deep learning in the context of medical decision support systems, and also importance of the diagnosis as followed more in this book.

After the start for essential concepts, it is better to deep inside in the next two chapters, by focusing on the widely known deep learning architectures, and then evaluating the literature including applications of deep learning architectures for medical diagnosis, as the decision support approach.

1.4 Further Learning

There are many more to discuss and express about artificial intelligence, and its roots as well as the associated topics. The interested readers in this manner are referred to [66–76] as some recent, and remarkable sources.

Currently, there are many different developments environment and even libraries for developing intelligent systems. The readers can read [77–85] in order to get some knowledge and skills about the widely used programming languages, and development perspectives.

For having some more information about decision support systems in general, the readers can read also the books [86–89].

References

1. I. McNeil (ed.), *An Encyclopedia of the History of Technology* (Routledge, 2002)
2. N. Rosenberg, R. Nathan, *Exploring the Black Box: Technology, Economics, and History* (Cambridge University Press, 1994)
3. D. Edgerton, *Shock of the Old: Technology and Global History Since 1900* (Profile Books, 2011)
4. M.R. Williams, *A History of Computing Technology* (IEEE Computer Society Press, 1997)

5. J.E. McClellan III, H. Dorn, *Science and Technology in World History: An Introduction* (JHU Press, 2015)
6. D.R. Headrick, *Technology: A World History* (Oxford University Press, 2009)
7. L. Rabelo, S. Bhide, E. Gutierrez, *Artificial Intelligence: Advances in Research and Applications* (Nova Science Publishers, Inc., 2018)
8. J. Romportl, E. Zackova, J. Kelemen, *Beyond Artificial Intelligence* (Springer International, 2016)
9. K. Henning, How artificial intelligence changes the world, in *Developing Support Technologies* (Springer, Cham, 2018), pp. 277–284
10. D. Tveter, *The Pattern Recognition Basis of Artificial Intelligence* (IEEE Press, 1997)
11. J.H. Holland, *Adaptation in Natural and Artificial Systems: An Introductory Analysis with Applications to Biology, Control, and Artificial Intelligence* (MIT Press, 1992)
12. J. Liebowitz, Knowledge management and its link to artificial intelligence. Expert Syst. Appl. **20**(1), 1–6 (2001)
13. C. Blum, R. Groß, Swarm intelligence in optimization and robotics, in *Springer Handbook of Computational Intelligence* (Springer, Berlin, Heidelberg, 2015), pp. 1291–1309
14. A. Pannu, Artificial intelligence and its application in different areas. Artif. Intell. **4**(10), 79–84 (2015)
15. Y. LeCun, Y. Bengio, G. Hinton, Deep learning. Nature **521**(7553), 436–444 (2015)
16. P. Ongsulee, Artificial intelligence, machine learning and deep learning, in *2017 15th International Conference on ICT and Knowledge Engineering (ICT&KE)* (IEEE, 2017), pp. 1–6
17. X. Du, Y. Cai, S. Wang, L. Zhang, Overview of deep learning, in *2016 31st Youth Academic Annual Conference of Chinese Association of Automation (YAC)* (IEEE, 2016), pp. 159–164
18. G. Nguyen, S. Dlugolinsky, M. Bobák, V. Tran, Á.L. García, I. Heredia, L. Hluchý, Machine learning and deep learning frameworks and libraries for large-scale data mining: a survey. Artif. Intell. Rev. **52**(1), 77–124 (2019)
19. D. Ravì, C. Wong, F. Deligianni, M. Berthelot, J. Andreu-Perez, B. Lo, G.Z. Yang, Deep learning for health informatics. IEEE J. Biomed. Health Inform. **21**(1), 4–21 (2016)
20. E. Alpaydin, *Introduction to Machine Learning* (MIT Press, 2020)
21. C. Xu, Y.C. Shin, *Intelligent Systems: Modeling, Optimization, and Control* (CRC Press, Inc., 2008)
22. M. Kppen, G. Schaefer, A. Abraham, *Intelligent Computational Optimization in Engineering: Techniques & Applications* (Springer Publishing Company, Incorporated, 2011)
23. O. Senvar, E. Turanoglu, C. Kahraman, Usage of metaheuristics in engineering: a literature review, in *Meta-Heuristics Optimization Algorithms in Engineering, Business, Economics, and Finance* (IGI Global, 2013), pp. 484–528
24. C.W. Kirkwood, *Strategic Decision Making* (Duxbury Press, 1997)
25. S. Plous, *The Psychology of Judgment and Decision Making* (Mcgraw-Hill Book Company, 1993)
26. E. Turban, *Decision Support and Expert Systems: Management Support Systems* (Prentice Hall PTR, 1993)
27. D.J. Power, *Decision Support Systems: Concepts and Resources for Managers* (Greenwood Publishing Group, 2002)
28. R.H. Bonczek, C.W. Holsapple, A.B. Whinston, *Foundations of Decision Support Systems* (Academic Press, 2014)
29. D. Power, Decision support systems: from the past to the future. AMCIS 2004 Proc. **242** (2004)
30. V. Rossi, T. Caffi, F. Salinari, Helping farmers face the increasing complexity of decision-making for crop protection. Phytopathol. Mediterr. 457–479 (2012)
31. C. Zopounidis, M. Doumpos, Developing a multicriteria decision support system for financial classification problems: the FINCLAS system. Optim. Methods Softw. **8**(3–4), 277–304 (1998)
32. C. Zopounidis, M. Doumpos, N.F. Matsatsinis, On the use of knowledge-based decision support systems in financial management: a survey. Decis. Support Syst. **20**(3), 259–277 (1997)
33. E. Tsang, P. Yung, J. Li, EDDIE-automation, a decision support tool for financial forecasting. Decis. Support Syst. **37**(4), 559–565 (2004)

34. H.J. von Mettenheim, M.H. Breitner, Robust decision support systems with matrix forecasts and shared layer perceptrons for finance and other applications, in *ICIS* (2010), p. 83
35. A. Asemi, A. Safari, A.A. Zavareh, The role of management information system (MIS) and decision support system (DSS) for manager's decision making process. Int. J. Bus. Manag. **6**(7), 164–173 (2011)
36. R. Sharda, S.H. Barr, J.C. MCDonnell, Decision support system effectiveness: a review and an empirical test. Manage. Sci. **34**(2), 139–159 (1988)
37. E.W. Ngai, F.K.T. Wat, Fuzzy decision support system for risk analysis in e-commerce development. Decis. Support Syst. **40**(2), 235–255 (2005)
38. V.L. Sauter, *Decision Support Systems for Business Intelligence* (Wiley, 2014)
39. K. Pal, O. Palmer, A decision-support system for business acquisitions. Decis. Support Syst. **27**(4), 411–429 (2000)
40. Y.K. Juan, P. Gao, J. Wang, A hybrid decision support system for sustainable office building renovation and energy performance improvement. Energy Build. **42**(3), 290–297 (2010)
41. D. Voivontas, D. Assimacopoulos, A. Mourelatos, J. Corominas, Evaluation of renewable energy potential using a GIS decision support system. Renew. Energy **13**(3), 333–344 (1998)
42. J.A. Cherni, I. Dyner, F. Henao, P. Jaramillo, R. Smith, R.O. Font, Energy supply for sustainable rural livelihoods. A multi-criteria decision-support system. Energy Policy **35**(3), 1493–1504 (2007)
43. A. Phdungsilp, Integrated energy and carbon modeling with a decision support system: policy scenarios for low-carbon city development in Bangkok. Energy Policy **38**(9), 4808–4817 (2010)
44. P. Zambelli, C. Lora, R. Spinelli, C. Tattoni, A. Vitti, P. Zatelli, M. Ciolli, A GIS decision support system for regional forest management to assess biomass availability for renewable energy production. Environ. Model Softw. **38**, 203–213 (2012)
45. S.B. Kotsiantis, Use of machine learning techniques for educational proposes: a decision support system for forecasting students' grades. Artif. Intell. Rev. **37**(4), 331–344 (2012)
46. W. Yahya, N. Noor, Decision support system for learning disabilities children in detecting visual-auditory-kinesthetic learning style, in *The 7th International Conference on Information Technology* (2015), pp. 667–671
47. H. Peng, P.Y. Chuang, G.J. Hwang, H.C. Chu, T.T. Wu, S.X. Huang, Ubiquitous performance-support system as mindtool: a case study of instructional decision making and learning assistant. J. Educ. Technol. Soc. **12**(1), 107–120 (2009)
48. P. Haastrup, V. Maniezzo, M. Mattarelli, F.M. Rinaldi, I. Mendes, M. Paruccini, A decision support system for urban waste management. Eur. J. Oper. Res. **109**(2), 330–341 (1998)
49. J. Coutinho-Rodrigues, A. Simão, C.H. Antunes, A GIS-based multicriteria spatial decision support system for planning urban infrastructures. Decis. Support Syst. **51**(3), 720–726 (2011)
50. S. Feng, L. Xu, An intelligent decision support system for fuzzy comprehensive evaluation of urban development. Expert Syst. Appl. **16**(1), 21–32 (1999)
51. H. Yan, Y. Jiang, J. Zheng, C. Peng, Q. Li, A multilayer perceptron-based medical decision support system for heart disease diagnosis. Expert Syst. Appl. **30**(2), 272–281 (2006)
52. D. West, V. West, Model selection for a medical diagnostic decision support system: a breast cancer detection case. Artif. Intell. Med. **20**(3), 183–204 (2000)
53. D.S. Kumar, G. Sathyadevi, S. Sivanesh, Decision support system for medical diagnosis using data mining. Int. J. Comput. Sci. Issues (IJCSI) **8**(3), 147 (2011)
54. E. Alickovic, A. Subasi, Medical decision support system for diagnosis of heart arrhythmia using DWT and random forests classifier. J. Med. Syst. **40**(4), 108 (2016)
55. M. Gaynor, M. Seltzer, S. Moulton, J. Freedman, A dynamic, data-driven, decision support system for emergency medical services, in *International Conference on Computational Science* (Springer, Berlin, Heidelberg, 2005), pp. 703–711
56. P.K. Anooj, Clinical decision support system: risk level prediction of heart disease using weighted fuzzy rules. J. King Saud Univ.-Comput. Inf. Sci. **24**(1), 27–40 (2012)
57. A. Subasi, Medical decision support system for diagnosis of neuromuscular disorders using DWT and fuzzy support vector machines. Comput. Biol. Med. **42**(8), 806–815 (2012)

58. R.A. Miller, Diagnostic decision support systems, in *Clinical Decision Support Systems* (Springer, Cham, 2016), pp. 181–208
59. V. Moret-Bonillo, I. Fernández-Varela, E. Hernández-Pereira, D. Alvarez-Estévez, V. Perlitz, On the automation of medical knowledge and medical decision support systems, in *Advances in Biomedical Informatics* (Springer, Cham, 2018), pp. 187–217
60. S. Belciug, F. Gorunescu, Intelligent systems and the healthcare revolution, in *Intelligent Decision Support Systems—A Journey to Smarter Healthcare* (Springer, Cham, 2020), pp. 259–266
61. S. Bashir, U. Qamar, F.H. Khan, L. Naseem, HMV: a medical decision support framework using multi-layer classifiers for disease prediction. J. Comput. Sci. **13**, 10–25 (2016)
62. H. Ltifi, M.B. Ayed, Visual intelligent decision support systems in the medical field: design and evaluation, in *Machine Learning for Health Informatics* (Springer, Cham, 2016), pp. 243–258
63. E.S. Kumar, P.S. Jayadev, Deep learning for clinical decision support systems: a review from the panorama of smart healthcare, in *Deep Learning Techniques for Biomedical and Health Informatics* (Springer, Cham, 2020), pp. 79–99
64. S. Spänig, A. Emberger-Klein, J.P. Sowa, A. Canbay, K. Menrad, D. Heider, The virtual doctor: an interactive clinical-decision-support system based on deep learning for non-invasive prediction of diabetes. Artif. Intell. Med. **100**, 101706 (2019)
65. J.T. Kim, Application of machine and deep learning algorithms in intelligent clinical decision support systems in healthcare. J. Health Med. Inform. **9**(05) (2018)
66. B.G. Buchanan, A (very) brief history of artificial intelligence. Ai Mag. **26**(4), 53 (2005)
67. N.J. Nilsson, *The Quest for Artificial Intelligence* (Cambridge University Press, 2009)
68. N. Ensmenger, Is chess the drosophila of artificial intelligence? A social history of an algorithm. Soc. Stud. Sci. **42**(1), 5–30 (2012)
69. S.L. Garfinkel, R.H. Grunspan, *The Computer Book: From the Abacus to Artificial Intelligence, 250 Milestones in the History of Computer Science* (Sterling Swift Pub Co, 2018)
70. M. Tegmark, *Life 3.0: Being Human in the Age of Artificial Intelligence* (Knopf, 2017)
71. A. Agrawal, J. Gans, A. Goldfarb, *Prediction Machines: The Simple Economics of Artificial Intelligence* (Harvard Business Press, 2018)
72. V.C. Müller, N. Bostrom, Future progress in artificial intelligence: a survey of expert opinion, in *Fundamental Issues of Artificial Intelligence* (Springer, Cham, 2016), pp. 555–572
73. I. Katsov, *Introduction to Algorithmic Marketing: Artificial Intelligence for Marketing Operations* (Ilia Katcov, 2017)
74. P. Joshi, *Artificial Intelligence with Python* (Packt Publishing Ltd, 2017)
75. F. Hutter, L. Kotthoff, J. Vanschoren, *Automated Machine Learning* (Springer, New York, NY, USA, 2019)
76. A. Menshawy, *Deep Learning By Example: A Hands-On Guide to Implementing Advanced Machine Learning Algorithms and Neural Networks* (Packt Publishing Ltd, 2018)
77. S. Raschka, *Python Machine Learning* (Packt Publishing Ltd, 2015)
78. J. Grus, *Data Science from Scratch: First Principles with Python* (O'Reilly Media, 2019)
79. S. Raschka, V. Mirjalili, *Python Machine Learning: Machine Learning and Deep Learning with Python, Scikit-Learn, and TensorFlow 2* (Packt Publishing Ltd, 2019)
80. J. Moolayil, S. John, *Learn Keras for Deep Neural Networks* (Apress, 2019)
81. J. Brownlee, *Deep Learning for Computer Vision: Image Classification, Object Detection, and Face Recognition in Python* (Machine Learning Mastery, 2019)
82. A. Paszke, S. Gross, F. Massa, A. Lerer, J. Bradbury, G. Chanan, A. Desmaison, PyTorch: an imperative style, high-performance deep learning library, in *Advances in Neural Information Processing Systems* (2019), pp. 8024–8035
83. M. Paluszek, S. Thomas, *MATLAB Machine Learning Recipes: A Problem-Solution Approach* (Apress, 2019)
84. J.V. Stone, *Artificial Intelligence Engines: A Tutorial Introduction to the Mathematics of Deep Learning* (Sebtel Press, 2019)
85. I. Livshin, *Artificial Neural Networks with Java* (Apress, 2019)

86. G.E. Kersten, Z Mikolajuk, A.G.O. Yeh, *Decision Support Systems for Sustainable Development: A Resource Book of Methods and Applications* (Springer Science & Business Media, 2000)
87. R. Sugumaran, J. Degroote, *Spatial Decision Support Systems: Principles and Practices* (CRC Press, 2010)
88. E. Lughofer, M. Sayed-Mouchaweh (eds.), *Predictive Maintenance in Dynamic Systems: Advanced Methods, Decision Support Tools and Real-World Applications* (Springer, 2019)
89. S. Latteman, *Development of an Environmental Impact Assessment and Decision Support System for Seawater Desalination Plants* (CRC Press, 2010)

Chapter 2
Deep Learning Architectures for Medical Diagnosis

Following an introduction to the artificial intelligence and decision support systems in the Chap. 1, it is possible to focus on deep learning and exact architectures of deep learning used for medical diagnosis.

As the technological developments are in a speedy rise, managing medical data and information is becoming a growing problem for healthcare professionals. A patient's health history includes a constantly growing set of data, such as medical data about his or her illnesses, diagnostic and treatment methods. The main problem in providing the necessary health services to the patients is to find and use the relevant information at the right time. For this purpose, some systems are designed to combine the necessary data such as general public health information, patient personal data, electronic healthcare records (EHR), medical reference books, web sites, research information and statistical reports designed specifically for consistent and reliable decisions and are called Clinical Decision Support Systems (CDSS). To answer the question of why CDSS are needed at every stage of the diagnosis and treatment of any medical disease for the decisions making, are of great importance. Health professionals' decision-making performance may be minimal and as complexity increases, the problem may worsen. Because of these, the development of a medical decision support system is gaining in importance and the use of these intelligent systems in all areas of medicine is increasingly common. The employment of artificial intelligence (AI) for ensuring medical decision-making accordingly is associated with the knowledge-intensive expert advisory systems introduced in the early 1970s. On the other hand, software environments with sophisticated features are in the trend of running AI approaches as well as methods together. Because they are also trying to facilitate the task of creating, verifying and testing their medical knowledge base. In short, CDSS is defined as an active intelligent system that can help medical professionals make specific decisions by taking specific recommendations. It also makes decisions based on the resolution of patient-specific information and relevant medical facts. These systems use AI methods, approaches, or techniques to make decisions.

U. Kose et al., *Deep Learning for Medical Decision Support Systems*, Studies in Computational Intelligence 909, https://doi.org/10.1007/978-981-15-6325-6_2

Fig. 2.1 Some medical tasks for CDSSs

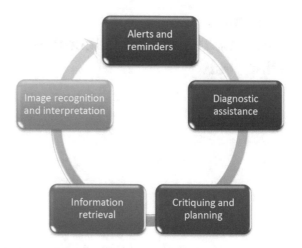

As shown in Fig. 2.1, CDSSs have been developed using artificial intelligence for many medical tasks to assist healthcare workers [1].

Almost every field of medicine has assistant software that uses AI methods. Recently, deep learning methods have been used for decision making in these software systems. In a general definition, deep learning is known as a sub-area of the machine learning. Here, higher-level concepts are defined rather than the concepts at lower-level so that it can help identifying still the same lower-level concepts, based on learning the various levels of representation corresponding to hierarchies of features or factors or concepts. In other words, the concept of deep learning is within the family of machine learning techniques, which are based on learning representations. At this point, it is possible to ensure observation representations via different ways, but some representations make it easier to learn related tasks from examples, and research in this field tries to define what is better represented and how to learn [2].

In is clearly seen recently, deep learning has been used in many fields of application and has been very successful. This new field of machine learning is growing rapidly and has been applied to most of the traditional application areas. Fast and efficient decision-making offers new opportunities for researchers. There are different solution ways as oriented on different approaches of learning: supervised, non-supervised, reinforcement, and also semi-supervised learning. Performed experimental applications point that they provide very good and efficient performance in many areas such as image processing, machine translation, computer vision, medical imaging, speech recognition, art, medical information processing, bioinformatics, robotics and control, natural language processing, cyber security etc. There are common methods in the field of Deep Learning (DL) starting from the Deep Neural Network (DNN). Also, Autoencoder Network (AEN), Deep Belief Network (DBN), Convolutional Neural Network (CNN), Recurrent Neural Network (RNN), Restricted Boltzmann Machine (RBM), and Deep Reinforcement Learning (DRL) are the most prominent DL methods. In addition, for good generalization, there are also improved autoencoder types such as stacked autoencoder (SAE) and denoising autoencoder (DAE).

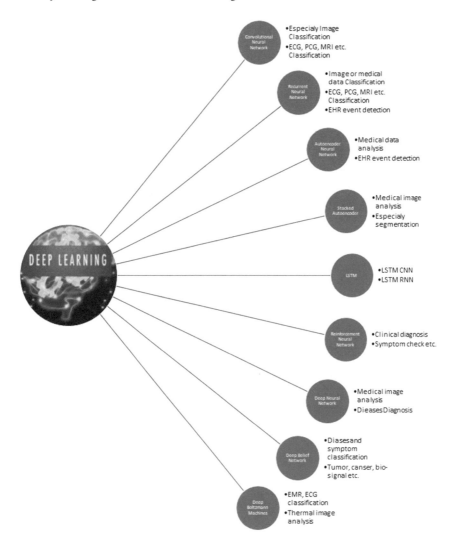

Fig. 2.2 Deep learning as used in the context of medical fields

Especially there are some DL techniques used in hybrid methods with CNN and RNN such as Long Short Term Memory (LSTM), and Gated recurrent units (GRUs) [3]. Naturally, deep learning has taken its place in many CDSSs in the medical field as well. They are particularly used in medical image processing (i.e. segmentation), computer vision, speech recognition (i.e. Parkinson's disease), medical imaging, medical information processing, and bioinformatics. Figure 2.2 represents the deep learning methods used in medical fields and the areas in which they are most used.

As seen in the figure, it is possible to come across many deep learning practices in almost every field of a medicine. The most widely employed one is the

Convolutional Neural Network with its superiority in image processing. A Recurrent Neural Network and an Autoencoder networks with hybrid methods followed the Convolutional Neural Network [4].

2.1 Deep Learning for Medical Diagnosis

Generally, the employment of deep learning within medical diagnostic procedures has two approaches for medical diagnostics. The first approach is used to process medical data or biomedical signals in databases. The second approach is used to process medical images. Example process steps for the first approach are given in Fig. 2.3.

In this type of diagnostic system, pre-processing is performed for incoming data. If the system entry is medical data from databases, are there missing data sets? Is controlled. Missing data is eliminated or new ones are added. If the input data is a biomedical signal, it is preprocessed according to the signal type. For example, for sound signals, first, the signals are digitized and prepared for resampling and normalization. Then resampling and normalization are performed. These preprocessing performed if necessary, after filtration the signals are ready for the diagnostic process. Finally, the classification process is performed with one of the deep learning methods to obtain a sample diagnosis estimate.

Example process steps for the second approach are given in Fig. 2.4. What makes the second approach different is that the input is a medical image. Of course, other signals whose images can be acquired can also be used as inputs. In this approach, first the sizes of the image are adjusted for image preprocessing. Then image enhancement operations are performed according to the type of image. These operations are mostly contrast enhancement, histogram equalization, contrast limited adaptive histogram

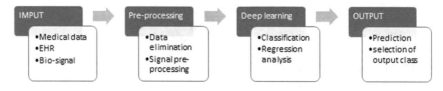

Fig. 2.3 The process steps for medical data or biomedical signal

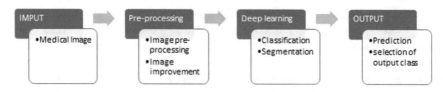

Fig. 2.4 The process steps for medical images or biomedical signal

equalization. Following these operations, filtering is performed to regulate colors or to adjust the edge sharpness. Mostly used filters are Gaussian, guided, homomorphic etc. Following image preprocessing, a segmentation of images for selection of objects or a classification is performed and deep learning according to this process is performed. After a segmentation, a classification is also performed for a prediction of any diseases.

As shown in both approach, appropriate preprocessing is performed for input data or images before applying the deep learning technique.

2.2 Deep Learning Architectures

In this section, the architectural structures of deep learning methods that are frequently used for medical diagnosis will be briefly discussed.

2.2.1 Convolutional Neural Networks

By far the most common use of parameter sharing in deep learning occurs in convolutional neural networks (CNN) applied to digital images. Natural images have many statistical features that do not change to translation. For example, a photo of a cat remains a photo of a cat if a pixel is turned to the right. CNNs take this feature into account by sharing parameters in multiple display locations. The same property is calculated at different positions in the input on a hidden unit with the same weights. In short, convolution is a special type of linear process. Convolutional networks are neural networks that use convolution instead of the general matrix product in at least one of its layers [5]. Figure 2.5 illustrates the basic structure of an example CNN. In the typical formation of the CNN, there are one or more convolution layers, and i.e. rectified linear unit (ReLU) layers, which are known as non-linear layers, and also Max-pooling layers. A typical CNN follows three steps as (1) a certain number of

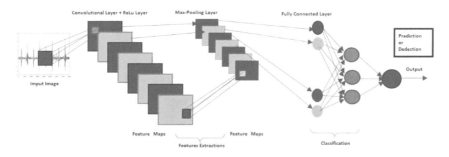

Fig. 2.5 The basic structure of an example CNN

folds for getting a series of linear activations, (2) linear activations done thanks to non-linear activation function like the rectified linear activation function (that is also called as the detector step), and finally (3) change over the output of the layer, with a pooling function accordingly used [2, 6].

To use highly correlated data sub regions, by calculating the convolutions between local patches and weight vectors called filters in each convolution layer, groups of local weighted totals are obtained at each convolution layer. Also, since the same models may be get as associated with the location in the data, the filters are applied to the entire data set repeatedly, as reducing the total number of parameters to be learned, thereby improving training efficiency. The nonlinear layers then increase the nonlinear properties of the feature maps. In each localization layer, maximum or average sub-sampling of non-overlapping regions in the feature maps is performed. That approach of overlapping subsampling enables a CNN to handle semantically similar but slightly different features, thus combining local features for identifying features in complex forms [6].

Finally, the classification is performed with fully connected neural network layers, typically tipped with a softmax layer that provides a probabilistic score for each class. Intuitively obvious, CNN encodes the input image with incremental abstraction as properties spread across network layers, resulting in an abstract classification option [7].

2.2.2   Recurrent Neural Networks

Recurrent neural networks (RNNs) are briefly a deep neural network model, which can be used with supervised or unsupervised learning. Here in detail, the depth to deal with can be as large as the length of the data sequence, which is used as the input. While in the mode of unsupervised learning, an RNN is used for predicting future series of data, thanks to previous data samples, and without needing additional classes information [2]. Figure 2.6 illustrates the basic structure of an example RNN. As

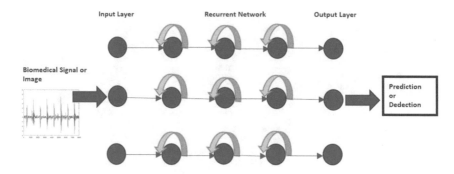

Fig. 2.6 The basic structure of an example RNN

can be seen from the figure, RNNs designed to use sequential information employs a simple structure with cyclic connection. Since the input data is processed sequentially, the repetitive calculation is performed in the hidden units with the cyclic connection. In detail, the historical information is stored in hidden units (in other terms, state vectors), and the output for current input is calculated using all of the previous inputs using the related state vectors [8]. Although RNNs attract less attention than DNNs and CNNs, they are among the most effective analysis methods against sequential information. Because omics data and biomedical signals are typically considered sequential and often natural languages, the ability of RNNs to match a variable length input sequence to another sequence or fixed-size prediction makes it ideal for bioinformatics research [6].

2.2.3 Autoencoder Neural Network

An autoencoder network (AEN) is a feedforward neural network that is trained to try to copy its input to its output. Figure 2.7 illustrates the basic structure of an example AEN.

The deep AEN is a special kind of deep learning without class label, the output vectors having the same dimensions as the input vectors. A typical AEN model is often used to learn a representation or running the task of effective encoding of the original data. AEN is a non-linear property extraction method without using class labels. Thus, even though these two objectives are sometimes associated,

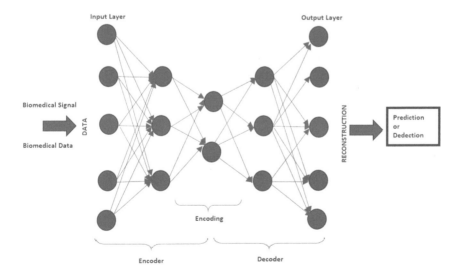

Fig. 2.7 The basic structure of an example AEN

the extracted features aim to preserve and better represent information rather than performing classification tasks [5].

As shown in the figure, an autoencoder typically runs an input layer, hidden layers, and then an output layer. First, it has an input layer representing the original data or input property vectors, such as pixels in the image or spectra in the speech. It is called an encoder with hidden layers. If the number of hidden layers is more than one, AEN is then considered as a deep neural network. It therefore has one or more hidden layers representing the transformed property. There is an output layer that matches the input layer for regenerating the encoded data. The output layer, together with hidden layers, is called a decoder. When the target property is compression, the size of hidden layers is smaller than the size of the input and output layers. Thus, AEN has a symmetrical structure. While the target property maps to a higher dimensional area, the size of the hidden layers is larger than the size of the input and output layers. The AEN structure is symmetrical in a decreasing structure from the inside out [5].

2.2.4   Deep Neural Networks

As can be seen in Fig. 2.8, the basic model formation of Deep Neural Networks (DNNs) includes respectively (1) an input layer, (2) multiple-hidden layers, and (3) an output layer. When input data is exported to DNNs, the output values are calculated sequentially along the network layers. In each layer, the input vector containing the output values of each unit in the following layer is multiplied by the weight vector of each unit in the current layer for getting the weighted layer. Next, a non-linear function like a hyperbolic tangent, sigmoid or a rectified linear unit (ReLU) is employed for calculating the output values corresponding to the layer. The calculation on each layer transforms the presentations on the following layer into slightly more abstract representations. It can be classified depending on the layer types used in the DNNs and the corresponding learning method [8, 9].

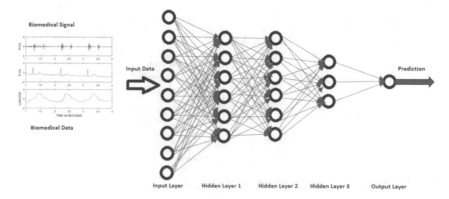

Fig. 2.8 The basic structure of an example DNN

It is possible to see a deep neural network model as a huge parallel distributed processor, which can learn and store experiential information. Information is acquired by the DNN system and then send through the structure of the model in the context of a learning process called as the machine self-learning capabilities. Interneuron connection forces, also known as weights in network system and architecture, are used to store information. During the training, a learning algorithm is used for the DNN classification model to change the weights of linear and nonlinear transfer functions within all neuron units in the network. In other words, the learning algorithm adjusts all weights of the DNN classification model according to the input data and output data of the target variable to achieve the best or better performance during each iterative process of the training sessions [10].

2.2.5 Deep Belief Network

Deep Belief Networks (DBNs) were one of the first non-evolutionary models developed by Hinton et al. [11]. Figure 2.9 provides an example DBN Structure with both routed and non-routed connections.

As such, it is like a Restricted Boltzmann Machines (RBM) but does not have inter-layer connections. In addition, a DBN can have multiple hidden layers. Therefore, the connections between the hidden units are on separate layers. All local conditional probability distributions required by the DBN are copied directly from the local conditional probability distributions of the constructor RBMs [5]. DBNs are graphical models that learn to generate a deep hierarchical representation of training data. DBNs are productive models that contain several hidden variable layers. While the apparent units can be binary or real, hidden variables are typically binary. There is no link between layers. Generally, each unit on each layer connects to each unit on each neighboring layer, but it is possible to create less frequently linked DBNs. Connections between the two layers in the input are not routed. Links between all other layers are oriented so that the arrows point to the layer closest to the data [12].

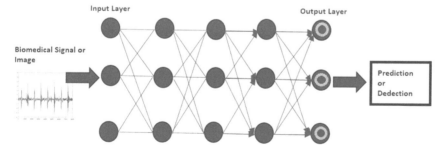

Fig. 2.9 The basic structure of an example DNN

2.2.6   Deep Reinforcement Learning

Deep Reinforcement Learning (DRL) is often recommended for applications that can interact with an environment and perform actions. DRL is a learning algorithm developed to train system parameters to interact and typically achieve specific goals. This learning algorithm can be realized by trial and error, demonstration or hybrid approach. As a representative takes action within his or her environment, a recurrent feedback loop of rewards and results trains the representative to better achieve the objectives at hand. Learning from the expert demonstration is accomplished either by learning to predict the actions of the experts through direct supervised learning or by subtracting the purpose of the expert. In order to successfully train a mediator, it is important to have a model function that can receive input signals from the medium as input senses and output subsequent actions for the mediator. DRL, where the deep learning model serves as a model function, is promising [13, 14].

2.2.7   Other Deep Learning Architectures

Out of the explained ones, the literature includes many more deep learning solutions used for a medical diagnostic. Less common DL methods than the above-mentioned of DL methods are briefly described below.

- Deep Boltzman Machine (DBM): DBM is a kind of binary Markov Random Field. This model is based on the Boltzmann family and consists of one-way connections between all hidden layers. In each layer, each of the variables is mutually independent, depending on the variables in adjacent layers. This model uses top-down feedback combined with ambiguous data and therefore provides robust inference. However, the training of a DBM is very costly in terms of calculation. Therefore, it is not possible to optimize the parameters for the large data set [4, 15].
- Stacked Auto-encoders: As the name implies, stacked auto-encoders, Denoising auto-encoders can be stacked to form a deep network by feeding the output code of the denoising autoencoder in the following layer as the input of the current layer. Here, while adding noise to the input, the network is expected to learn to distinguish between real and noisy signals. Unsupervised pre-training is carried out in one layer at a time. Each layer input, which is the exit code of the previous layer, is trained as a denoising autoencoder, minimizing the error while reconfiguring the input. Such an architecture becomes even more important in the case of medical data sets where noise is inherently present and the cleaning of such datasets is not only expensive, but subjective [4, 12].
- Different methods have been tried to solve the learning problems of RNN in particular. For example, gated recurrent neural networks have begun to be taken into account during numerical gradient calculation. Two commonly used methods for CNN and RNN are Gated recurrent units (GRUs) and long short term memory

(LSTM). The difficulty of addressing long-term information protection and short-term input skipping in hidden variable models has long been the subject of research. Hochreiter and Schmidhuber proposed the LSTM approach for this. There are many common features between GRU and LSTM. The GRU approach was developed before LSTM and has a slightly simpler structure [13, 16].

- LSTM is a type of network that uses special hidden volumes that are natural to remember entries for a long time. A special unit called a memory cell acts as an accumulator or a gated leaky neuron: it has a connection with a weight next time. Therefore, it copies its true value and accumulates the external signal. However, this self-connection is multiplied by another unit that learns to decide when to clear the contents of the memory. LSTM and RNN hybrid networks have proven to be more effective than normal RNNs. In particular, when they have several layers for each time step, they provide a complete speech recognition system, ranging from acoustic to transcribed character strings. LSTM networks or related forms of related units are also currently used for encoder and decoder networks which perform very well in machine translation [8].

2.3 Summary

For the past fifteen years, there have been many deep learning methods used for medical diagnostics. It is frequently used in medical image processing (i.e. segmentation), computer vision, speech recognition (i.e. Parkinson's disease), medical imaging, medical information processing, and bioinformatics. There are common methods in the field of Deep Learning (DL) for a medical task starting from the Deep Neural Network (DNN). Also, Autoencoder Network (AEN), Deep Belief Network (DBN), Convolutional Neural Network (CNN), Recurrent Neural Network (RNN), Restricted Boltzmann Machine (RBM), and Deep Reinforcement Learning (DRL) are the most prominent DL methods. In addition, for good generalization, there are also improved autoencoder types such as stacked auto encoder (SAE) and denoising autoencoder (DAE). Especially there are some DL techniques used in hybrid methods with CNN and RNN such as Long Short Term Memory (LSTM), and Door Repeating Units (GRU).

There are many deep learning practices in almost every field of medicine. The most common and the most preferred is the Convolution Neural Network, which has superiority in image processing. Recurrent Neural Network and Autoencoder networks follow Convolutional Neural Network with improved versions and hybrid methods.

After explaining essentials of the widely used deep learning architectures in medical applications, the literature can be examined in detail for understanding which kind of research is currently done by considering deep learning architectures. The following Chap. 3 provides a general view in this manner.

2.4   Further Learning

In order to see in detail, the characteristics of deep learning techniques and methods, readers are referred to [2–5, 8, 12, 13, 17].

From the studies, basics of DL methods and applications of different methods of DL in health care categorized as biological system, electronic health record, medical image and physiological signals, the basics of DL methods and areas where medical DL applications are widely used can be seen [18, 19].

The use of DL methods in medical diagnostics can be explored in order to obtain detailed information in [4, 6, 14, 17, 20–30].

Those who want to do detailed research in medical image processing, classification and diagnostic procedures, especially CNN, can look at the examples given in [7, 31, 32].

The scientists who want to learn how to reach dataset to diagnose different types of cancer with deep learning, can examine [33]. Also, they can find which proposed methods for this, public databases commonly used in these methods.

The readers looking for a review of deep learning techniques for health care in natural language processing, computer vision, reinforcing learning, and generalized methods, also can read [34–39].

For the most recent developments reported in the context of highly reputable journals, the readers are referred to [14, 40–51].

References

1. O. Deperlioglu, Intelligent techniques inspired by nature and used in biomedical engineering, in *Biotechnology: Concepts, Methodologies, Tools, and Applications* (IGI Global, 2019), pp. 666–692
2. L. Deng, D. Yu, Deep learning: methods and applications. Foundations Trends® Sig. Process. **7**(3–4), 197–387 (2014)
3. M.Z. Alom, T.M. Taha, C. Yakopcic, S. Westberg, P. Sidike, M.S. Nasrin, V.K. Asari, A state-of-the-art survey on deep learning theory and architectures. Electronics **8**(3), 292 (2019)
4. S. Srivastava, S. Soman, A. Rai, P.K. Srivastava, Deep learning for health informatics: recent trends and future directions, in *2017 International Conference on Advances in Computing, Communications and Informatics (ICACCI)*. (IEEE, 2017), pp. 1665–1670
5. I. Goodfellow, Y. Bengio, A. Courville, *Deep Learning* (MIT Press, 2016)
6. S. Min, B. Lee, S. Yoon, Deep learning in bioinformatics. Brief. Bioinform. **18**(5), 851–869 (2017)
7. L. Lu, Y. Zheng, G. Carneiro, L. Yang, Deep learning and convolutional neural networks for medical image computing, in *Advances in Computer Vision and Pattern Recognition* (Springer: New York, 2017)
8. Y. LeCun, Y. Bengio, G. Hinton, Deep learning. Nature **521**(7553), 436–444 (2015)
9. V. Nair, G.E. Hinton, Rectified linear units improve restricted Boltzmann machines, in *Proceedings of the 27th international conference on machine learning (ICML-10)* (2010), pp. 807–814
10. K.H. Miaao, J.H. Miaao, Coronary heart disease diagnosis using deep neural networks. Int. J. Adv. Comput. Sci. Appl. **9**(10), 1–8 (2018)
11. G.E. Hinton, S. Osindero, Y.W. Teh, A fast learning algorithm for deep belief nets. Neural Comput. **18**(7), 1527–1554 (2006)

12. Tutorial, *Deep Learning*. Release 0.1, LISA Lab (University of Montreal, 2015)
13. A. Zhang, Z.C. Lipton, M. Li, A.J. Smola, *Dive into Deep Learning*. Unpublished draft. Retrieved, 3, 319 (2019)
14. A. Esteva, A. Robicquet, B. Ramsundar, V. Kuleshov, M. DePristo, K. Chou, C. Cui, G. Corrado, J. Dean, A guide to deep learning in healthcare. Nat. Med. **25**(1), 24–29 (2019)
15. G. Litjens, T. Kooi, B.E. Bejnordi, A.A.A. Setio, F. Ciompi, M. Ghafoorian, J.A. Van Der Laak, C.I. Sánchez, A survey on deep learning in medical image analysis. Med. Image Anal., **42**, 60–88 (2017)
16. S. Hochreiter, J. Schmidhuber, Long short-term memory. Neural Comput. **9**(8), 1735–1780 (1997)
17. A.S. Bist, A survey of deep learning algorithms for malware detection. Int. J. Comput. Sci. Inf. Secur. (IJCSIS), **16**(3) (2018)
18. I. Tobore, J. Li, L. Yuhang, Y. Al-Handarish, A. Kandwal, Z. Nie, L. Wang, Deep learning intervention for health care challenges: some biomedical domain considerations. JMIR mHealth uHealth **7**(8), e11966 (2019)
19. A. Kandwal, Z. Nie, L. Wang, Deep learning intervention for health care challenges: some biomedical domain considerations
20. A. Jonsson, Deep reinforcement learning in medicine. Kidney Dis. **5**(1), 18–22 (2019)
21. A. Rajkomar, E. Oren, K. Chen, A.M. Dai, N. Hajaj, M. Hardt, M. Hardt, P.J. Liu, X. Liu, M. Sun, Sundberg, P, Scalable and accurate deep learning with electronic health records. NPJ Digit. Med. **1**(1), 18 (2018)
22. O. Gottesman, F. Johansson, M. Komorowski, A. Faisal, D. Sontag, F. Doshi-Velez, L.A. Celi, Guidelines for reinforcement learning in healthcare. Nat. Med. **25**(1), 16–18 (2019)
23. C. Wu, C. Luo, N. Xiong, W. Zhang, T.H. Kim, A greedy deep learning method for medical disease analysis. IEEE Access **6**, 20021–20030 (2018)
24. T. Davenport, R. Kalakota, The potential for artificial intelligence in healthcare. Future Healthc. J. **6**(2), 94–98 (2019)
25. M. Fatima, M. Pasha, Survey of machine learning algorithms for disease diagnostic. J. Intell. Learn. Syst. Appl. **9**(01), 1 (2017)
26. A. Rajkomar, J. Dean, I. Kohane, Machine learning in medicine. N. Engl. J. Med. **380**(14), 1347–1358 (2019)
27. F. Wang, A. Preininger, AI in health: state of the art, challenges, and future directions. Yearb. Med. Inform. **28**(01), 016–026 (2019)
28. C. Krittanawong, K.W. Johnson, R.S. Rosenson, Z. Wang, M. Aydar, U. Baber, J.K. Mun, W.W. Tang, J.L. Halperin, S.M. Narayan, Deep learning for cardiovascular medicine: a practical primer. Eur. Heart J. (2019)
29. A. Kassam, N. Kassam, Artificial intelligence in healthcare: a Canadian context, in *Healthcare Management Forum*, Vol. 33(1). (Sage Publications, Sage: Los Angeles, 2019), pp. 5–9
30. J. Mason, S. Visintini, T. Quay, An overview of clinical applications of 3-D printing and bioprinting, in *CADTH Issues in Emerging Health Technologies* (Canadian Agency for Drugs and Technologies in Health, 2019)
31. A.S. Lundervold, A. Lundervold, An overview of deep learning in medical imaging focusing on MRI. Z. für Med. Phys. **29**(2), 102–127 (2019)
32. J. Gao, Q. Jiang, B. Zhou, D. Chen, Convolutional neural networks for computer-aided detection or diagnosis in medical image analysis: an overview. Math. Biosci. Eng. **16**(6), 6536 (2019)
33. K. Munir, H. Elahi, A. Ayub, F. Frezza, A. Rizzi, Cancer diagnosis using deep learning: a bibliographic review. Cancers **11**(9), 1235 (2019)
34. K. Suzuki, Overview of deep learning in medical imaging. Radiol. Phys. Technol. **10**(3), 257–273 (2017)
35. S.K. Zhou, H. Greenspan, D. Shen, (Eds.) *Deep Learning for Medical Image Analysis* (Academic Press, 2017)
36. S. Bacchi, L. Oakden-Rayner, T. Zerner, T. Kleinig, S. Patel, J. Jannes, Deep learning natural language processing successfully predicts the cerebrovascular cause of transient ischemic attack-like presentations. Stroke **50**(3), 758–760 (2019)

37. Q. Chen, J. Du, S. Kim, W.J. Wilbur, Z. Lu, Combining rich features and deep learning for finding similar sentences in electronic medical records, in *Proceedings of the BioCreative/OHNLP Challenge*, 5–8 (2018)
38. R. Miotto, F. Wang, S. Wang, X. Jiang, J.T. Dudley, Deep learning for healthcare: review, opportunities and challenges. Brief. Bioinform. **19**(6), 1236–1246 (2018)
39. O. Faust, Y. Hagiwara, T.J. Hong, O.S. Lih, U.R. Acharya, Deep learning for healthcare applications based on physiological signals: a review. Comput. Methods Progr. Biomed. **161**, 1–13 (2018)
40. K.H. Yu, A.L. Beam, I.S. Kohane, Artificial intelligence in healthcare. Nat. Biomed. Eng. **2**(10), 719–731 (2018)
41. M. Alloghani, T. Baker, D. Al-Jumeily, A. Hussain, J. Mustafina, A.J. Aljaaf, Prospects of machine and deep learning in analysis of vital signs for the improvement of healthcare services, in *Nature-Inspired Computation in Data Mining and Machine Learning* (Springer, Cham, 2020), pp. 113–136
42. H. Lee, S. Yune, M. Mansouri, M. Kim, S.H. Tajmir, C.E. Guerrier, S.A. Ebert, S.R. Pomerantz, J.M. Kamalian, R.G. Gonzalez, An explainable deep-learning algorithm for the detection of acute intracranial haemorrhage from small datasets. Nat. Biomed. Eng., **3**(3), 173 (2019)
43. M.I. Jordan, T.M. Mitchell, Machine learning: trends, perspectives, and prospects. Science **349**(6245), 255–260 (2015)
44. S.G. Finlayson, J.D. Bowers, J. Ito, J.L. Zittrain, A.L. Beam, I.S. Kohane, Adversarial attacks on medical machine learning. Science **363**(6433), 1287–1289 (2019)
45. B. Sanchez-Lengeling, A. Aspuru-Guzik, Inverse molecular design using machine learning: generative models for matter engineering. Science **361**(6400), 360–365 (2018)
46. A. Mincholé, B. Rodriguez, Artificial intelligence for the electrocardiogram. Nat. Med. **25**(1), 22–23 (2019)
47. D.S. Kermany, M. Goldbaum, W. Cai, C.C. Valentim, H. Liang, S.L. Baxter, A. McKeown, G. Yang, X. Wu, F. Yan, J. Dong, Identifying medical diagnoses and treatable diseases by image-based deep learning. Cell, **172**(5), 1122–1131 (2018)
48. M. Koch, Artificial intelligence is becoming natural. Cell **173**(3), 533 (2018)
49. B. Norgeot, B.S. Glicksberg, L. Trupin, D. Lituiev, M. Gianfrancesco, B. Oskotsky, G. Schmajuk, J. Yazdany, A.J. Butte, Assessment of a deep learning model based on electronic health record data to forecast clinical outcomes in patients with rheumatoid arthritis. JAMA Netw. Open **2**(3), e190606–e190606 (2019)
50. F. Wang, L.P. Casalino, D. Khullar, Deep learning in medicine—promise, progress, and challenges. JAMA Intern. Med. **179**(3), 293–294 (2019)
51. A.D. Trister, The tipping point for deep learning in oncology. JAMA Oncol. **5**(10), 1429–1430 (2019)

Chapter 3
A Brief View on Medical Diagnosis Applications with Deep Learning

It is thought that deep learning will be more effective in the near future and will be used more in medical applications. Because it does not require too many input parameters and users do not need to have expert knowledge. In addition, it is not affected by the increases in the amount of calculation and data, and responds faster than traditional methods. Continuous improvement and development in the field of deep learning will also contribute to this process. That is because of highly advanced and flexible architectures of the deep learning as well as remarkable advantages as listed in Fig. 3.1. It is remarkable that the feature of flexibility has been always a critical advantage of artificial intelligence so that it has been applied to different fields. That has been seen in especially machine learning algorithms—techniques, thanks to the learning mechanism from data sets. As the deep learning is the advanced form of the machine learning, deep learning architectures have that flexibility, too. Moving from that, the architectures of the deep learning are widely used for different medical problems.

It is important that even medical diagnosis include many sub-problems having different difficulty levels. In this chapter, some recent and remarkable applications of the deep learning architectures—methods used in medical diagnostics (as expressed in the previous Chap. 2) for common areas are explained accordingly.

3.1 Convolutional Neural Networks Applications

Since CNNs are developed especially for processing 2D images, it is a commonly used method for the classification of medical images and diagnosing diseases from images. Therefore, it is one of the most widely used deep learning methods in the medical field. Some CNN applications used in medical diagnosis are given below.

Bakator and Radosavun conducted a comprehensive analysis of articles using deep neural networks in the medical field. They reviewed more than 300 research

U. Kose et al., *Deep Learning for Medical Decision Support Systems*, Studies in Computational Intelligence 909, https://doi.org/10.1007/978-981-15-6325-6_3

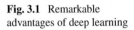

Fig. 3.1 Remarkable advantages of deep learning

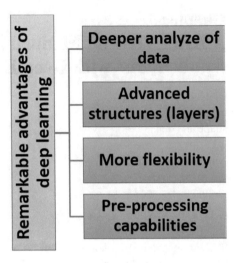

articles, including 46 articles in detail. Consequently, they found that CNN are the most widely used when it comes to deep learning and medical image analysis. They indicated that CNN are used to classify, and segment and automatic localize for many medical images such as computed tomography (CT), Fundus images, Mammography, Magnetic resonance imaging (MRI), Electrocardiogram (ECG) [1]. Neelapu et al. used CNN to classify medical images. They made a comparison for this method with two classical models such as Support vector machine (SVM), and extraordinary learning machine (ELM). According to their results, CNN is better than SVM and ELM in the classification of medical images [2].

In his study, Deperlioglu classified CNN as segmented and non-segmented Phonocardiograms (PCG) obtained from heart sounds in PASCAL and PhysioNet databases. Thus, he tried to diagnose heart diseases such as extrasystole and murmur. In this study, it was stated that conventional neural networks obtained better results than artificial neural network (ANN) for classification accuracy rate [3, 4]. Fujita and Cimr proposed a computer aided diagnosis system to diagnosis heart diseases such as fibrillations and flutters. This system only uses normalization and feature extraction from raw ECG images and uses CNN for classification [5]. Hemant and his colleagues attempted to diagnose diabetic retinopathy from color retinal fundus images in the Messidor database. For this purpose, they improved the fundus images with contrast limited adaptive histogram equalization method and classified them with CNN [6]. In their study, Deperlioglu and Kose proposed a method which contains an image processing method with HSV-V transform technique and a classification with CNN to diagnose diabetic retinopathy from color retinal fundus images in the Kaggle database [7]. All of them emphasized that CNN is an ideal classifier and very effective in the diagnosis of heart disease by the classification of PCGs.

In another study using image processing and CNN, Alfonso and his colleagues tried to diagnose Parkinson's disease. First, some specific drawings were made to the diseased and healthy individuals and the signals were recorded. The signals were transferred to the images by means of the iteration graph method, whose outputs emphasize the patterns of each class. The classification was then performed using a CNN. They emphasized that CNN is an ideal classifier and very effective in the diagnosis of Parkinson's disease from the brain signals [8]. Längkvist et al. tried to diagnose ureteral stones by classifying computed tomography (CT) images with CNN. They have proposed the use of CNN that directly processes high-resolution CT images to overcome the difficulty in effectively dealing with the similarity in shape and density of non-stone structures in urinary stones and large high-resolution CT volumes. They emphasized that they achieved very good results [9]. Iqbal and his colleagues suggested CNN to segment brain tumors on MRIs. To test the performance of the proposed method, they used the BRATS segmentation test data set consisting of images obtained by four different methods. From the experimental results on the BRATS 2015 comparison data, they demonstrated the usability of the proposed approach and its superiority over other approaches in this research area [10]. In order to recognize body parts, Yan and colleagues first conducted learning with CNN to remove the most discriminatory and non-informative local patches from the training slices. In the support phase, the previously learned CNN is further strengthened by these local patches for image classification. The main feature of the method is the selection of the body part with the actual information by automatically eliminating local and non-discriminatory patches through multi-sample deep learning. Thus, it can automatically identify from outside without any intervention [11].

Bar et al. examined the performance of CNN for pathology detection in chest radiography data. They investigated the ability of a CNN to identify different pathologies on chest X-ray images and the feasibility of using the same study in non-medical data [12]. Okomato et al. proposed a method for detecting hepatocellular carcinoma, namely liver cancer, by classifying CT images by CNN. By classifying a total of 1200 CT images in DICOM format with CNN, the validity and usefulness of the diagnostic procedure with CNN has been proven [13]. A study was carried out to determine the optimal size of the training dataset required to achieve high classification accuracy with low variance in medical image classification systems using another CT and CNN. By classification with CNN, axial CT images were divided into six anatomical classes. They trained CNN using six different sizes of training data sets (5, 10, 20, 50, 100 and 200) and tested the resulting system with a total of 6000 CT images. All images are in PACS format. The article focuses on the optimization of the data set size to obtain best classification accuracy [14].

There are many studies conducted with CNN for different diseases that cannot be mentioned here. Here are just a few applications done in recent years for different topics. As can be seen from the given applications, CNNs are often used for the processing and classification of medical images. In other words, CNNs or hybrid CNNs are thought that they are the first solutions that come to a scientist mind for a computer-assisted diagnostic system to be created by evaluating medical images.

3.2   Recurrent Neural Networks Applications

Recently, RNN has been used successfully in speech recognition, character recognition and many other AI tasks. However, this model has many difficulties due to its gradient disappearance and needs large data sets. Although RNNs have not improved as much as DNNs and CNNs, they still provide very powerful analysis methods for sequential information. Since omics data and biomedical signals can be processed as time series, the ability of RNNs to match a variable-length input sequence to another sequence or fixed-size estimation makes it readily available in bioinformatics research. It is believed that the proliferation of dynamic CT and MRI will enhance the long-term importance of RNNs, although RNNs are not currently preferred as CNNs in biomedical image processing. In addition, it is thought that their success in natural language processing may be more effective than the application of RNNs in biomedical text analysis and bioinformatics data [15, 16]. Some medical diagnostic applications with RNN are given below.

Guler et al. evaluated the diagnostic accuracy by classifying Lyapunov bases trained on the electroencephalogram (EEG) signals by the Levenberg-Marquardt algorithm with RNN. Elman RNNs designed and trained together with Lyapunov bases have proposed a method to diagnose epileptic seizures of EEG signals. In this study, it was stated that RNNs obtained higher accuracy rates than feed-forward neural network models [17]. In her article, Ubeyli made applications with different classification algorithms and compared classification accuracy rates in order to develop an automatic decision support system for breast cancer detection. These classifiers are multilayer sensor neural network (MLPNN), combined neural network (CNN), probability neural network (PNN), repetitive neural network (RNN) and support vector machine (SVM). In his research using the Wisconsin breast cancer database, SVM gave the best accuracy in diagnosis [18]. Al-Askar et al. have tested with different RNNs to demonstrate that RNNs such as the Elman network show significant improvements when used for pattern recognition in medical time series data analysis and achieve high accuracy in the classification of medical signals. For this purpose, a case study using Elman, Jordan and Layer recurrent networks for the classification of uterine electrohysterography signals for term and prediction of preterm birth of pregnant women is also presented. Efficiency of Elman RNN was tried to be shown [19].

Historical electronic health records (EHR) data consist of series of visits over time for each patient, including multiple medical codes, including diagnosis, medication, and patient profile at each visit. Using historical data from the EHR, the patient's medical conditions and drug use can be predicted of possible symptoms. Mu et al. classified EHR data using RNN. However, they proposed the use of bi-directional RNNs to remember all the information of both past and future visits and to add some patient characteristics as side information to this model. Their results show that the diagnosis of diseases from EHR datasets with the proposed model can significantly improve prediction accuracy and provide clinically meaningful interpretation compared to previous diagnostic prediction approaches [20]. In another study to estimate using large historical data EHRs, Choi et al., developed a generic estimation system covering observed medical conditions, and drug use. The system was called Doctor AI. The doctor AI was designed as a temporary system using RNN and tested with EHR data covering an 8-year time interval for 260,000 patients and 2128 physicians. In this study, RNN was used to estimate diagnostic and drug categories for a subsequent visit with diagnostic records, drug codes, or procedure codes examination records. At the end of the test, they claimed that Doctor AI could be generalized by adapting it from one organization to another without compromising accuracy [21]. In a similar study for prediction from EHRs, Jagannatha and Yu used Bidirectional RNN for prediction [22].

Transcranial Doppler (TCD) is a noninvasive technique for the diagnosis of cerebrovascular diseases using blood flow velocity measurements of cerebral artery segments. Seera et al. classified the features extracted from TCD signals using a series of RNN models with recurrent feedback. In addition to the individual RNN results, they established a community RNN model using majority voting to combine individual RNN estimates into an integrated estimate. The results showed that the RNN population is an effective method for detecting and classifying blood flow rate changes due to brain diseases [23]. Szkoła and his colleagues have developed a computer-based clinical decision support system (CDSS) for diagnosis laryngopathies. In their study, RNN was used for pattern recognition by accepting time series data in speech signals in the proposed CDSS. Thus, they analyzed speech signals using RNN. Validation experiments were performed on the speech signals of the patients in the control group with two groups of laryngopathy. A hybrid RNN consisting of Elman nets and Jordan nets was used. Modified Elman-Jordan networks show a faster and more accurate success of the target pattern [24].

Just as in CNNs, many more medical diagnostics applications can be given for RNNs. As can be seen from the given applications, RNNs are generally one of the most preferred methods for time series solutions. In this context, it is used for the processing and classification of all medical signals that can be considered as natural language analysis or time series expansion. In other words, RNNs or hybrid RNNs are the first solutions that come to mind for a computer-assisted diagnostic system to obtain an optimal prediction by evaluating medical signals (such as ECG, PCG, EEG) or data that may vary greatly over time (i.e. EHR).

3.3 Autoencoder Neural Network Applications

The problem of classification of unbalanced data has always been an important research topic in the field of machine learning. Autoencoder (AE) is a neural network that has specific capabilities to overcome these challenges in deep neural networks. When synthesizing new minority class samples, the over-sampling algorithm has the ability to respond to over-fitting and noise problems. The abundance of data in medical diagnostics and the fact that they have very different unique characteristics show that an autoencoder deep neural networks are very suitable for this area. Some medical diagnostic applications using an autoencoder are given below.

Deperlioglu used the main components of heart sounds, segmentation of S1-S2 sounds, and autoencoder, one of the deep learning methods to make high performance classification. In the study, first S1-S2 segmented heart sounds, then autoencoder neural network was used to classify these segmented sounds. He used the commonly used PASCAL B-training heart sounds data set to assess classification success. The results obtained in the classification study showed that the AEN gave better results than the feedforward artificial neural networks and other traditional methods [25]. Biomedical decision support systems have been developed in order to make better use of available data and assist doctors in the medical diagnosis and treatment phase. The most important component of biomedical decision support systems is the classification process that evaluates and compares the available data [26]. Deperlioglu has shown in a series of studies that the efficiency of AEN increases the success of BDSS. In these studies, generally well-known and publicly available medical databases were used to evaluate the performance of the autoencoder. The used datasets are Wisconsin Breast Cancer, and Hepatitis which are commonly used from medical datasets at the University of California Irvine (UCI) machine learning laboratory. The results of the studies showed that the accuracy, sensitivity and specificity values obtained by autoencoder were much higher than the artificial neural networks (ANN) that learned with Bayes regularization algorithm which performed with the same medical databases and gave the best classification success in [26]. It has also shown that it has a higher performance than previous traditional methods [25, 27, 28].

In their study, Arifoglu and Bouchachia used an AEN to exclude characteristics of image blocks that exhibited low coding errors. They examined the histogram of the automatic coding errors of the image blocks for each image class in order to decide which image regions or what percentage of an image would be considered the relevant area of interest. To validate the proposed scheme, they used local binary patterns (LBP) and support vector machines (SVM). They used the IRMA dataset with 14,410 X-ray images as the test data. They stated that this method can accelerate more than 27% in accuracy with a cost of less than 1% [29].

In an article on the classification of lung nodule images for the early diagnosis of lung cancer, the AEN network and softmax algorithm were used. First, lung nodule images were subdivided into local segments with Superpixel and then transformed into fixed length local feature vectors using an AEN. Based on these features, visual vocabulary was created. A visual bag of words was used to represent the characteristics of the lung nodule image. Finally, the softmax algorithm was used to classify the properties. Performance evaluation of the proposed method was performed using the publicly available and widely used ELCAP lung image database. It is stated that the proposed method is very efficient in terms of accuracy, sensitivity and specificity [30]. The AEN can also be used as a hybrid to solve the labeled data set problem in the CNN. For example, due to privacy and security issues, it is a major challenge to create a sufficiently labeled data set for CT analysis. Therefore, a convolutional automatic encoder is proposed to support the learned uncontrolled image properties for the lung nodule through unlabeled data that requires only a small amount of labeled data for effective feature learning. In the evaluations, they showed superiority over other methods and the convolutional auto-encoder approach proposed for the measurement of similarity of lung nodules could be extended [31].

As can be seen from the given applications, AENs are generally one of the most preferred methods for large numerical data or statistical analysis. In this context, it is used for the processing and classification of all medical signals or medical data, which can be obtained with equal weighted features (i.e. features vectors or matrices). In other words, AENs or enhanced AENs are the first solutions that come to mind for a computer-assisted diagnostic system to be created by evaluating medical signals (such as ECG, PCG, EEG) or very large data.

3.4 Deep Neural Network Applications

DNNs are widely used for high-dimensional and complex analysis and evaluation as in Bioinformatics data. The future progression of DNNs in bioinformatics can make it one of the most convenient ways to encode raw data from research and learn the appropriate properties from them [15].

Medical diagnostic systems based on deep learning can achieve diagnostic performance comparable to physicians in various medical use situations for many diseases. To be useful in practical applications in the clinic, it is necessary to have well-adjusted measurements of the uncertainty in which these systems report their decisions. However, deep neural networks (DNNs) often rely heavily on their estimates and are not suitable for direct probable treatment. To overcome this, Ayhan et al. proposed an intuitive framework based on test-time data enhancement to measure the diagnostic uncertainty of a DNN for the diagnosis of diabetic retinopathy [32]. Leibig et al. have proposed a method that uses DNN to diagnose diabetic retinopathy from digital color fundus images. They used Kaggle diabetic retinopathy dataset to test the proposed method. Apart from an efficient diagnosis, this study has shown that decision guidance with uncertainty information can improve diagnostic performance and generalize in different tasks and datasets [33]. In addition, DNN is used inside for vascular segmentation in color retinal images. Li et al. proposed a DNN-containing approach for vascular segmentation in retinal images. The proposed network can automatically learn the vascular feature in the training procedure. They showed that the proposed network is broad, and deep and has a stronger ability for induction than other conventional neural networks. The network can directly map the label of all pixels in a given image. In the estimation process, each pixel can be supported by more than one neighborhood and reduces image noise and uncertainty of pathology compared to one-off prediction [34]. Early diagnosis of heart diseases with deep learning methods. Miao et al. conducted a study to improve the accuracy and reliability of heart disease diagnosis and prognosis in patients using a DNN. In this method, they used a deep multilayered DNN learning model with regularization and release using deep learning. They used the data set of 303 clinical cases from patients diagnosed with coronary heart disease at the Cleveland Clinic Foundation as training data to test the proposed model and to identify potential new patients. The recommended medical diagnostic system for heart diseases is reported to be very efficient [35]. Agravat and Raval performed segmentation of tumors in the brain using MRI images and DNN. Any of the four MRI methods, i.e., T1, T2, T1c and FLAIR images, are provided as input to a tumor-degrading method. They tested the proposed method with public data. They said that deep neural networks had the ability to find an excellent automatic feature and that they were fighting the curse of dimensionality [36]. In another image processing study, Cireşan et al. used deep maximum pooled meandering neural networks to detect mitosis in breast histology images. In this study, using DNN as a pixel classifier for feature selection, they have pointed out the advantages of DNN in pixel classification [37].

In another study, a lung cancer diagnostic system based on Deep Learning was proposed. The proposed system classifies with DNN using data obtained from human urine by Gas Chromatography Mass Spectrometry (GC-MS). The proposed method has achieved 90% accuracy in assessing whether the patient has lung cancer. It was stated that this system would be useful for early diagnosis [38].

As can be seen from the applications given, although DNNs are generally one of the preferred methods for very large complex medical data or statistical analysis, they can be also used in medical image processing and a segmentation of medical images or a selection of image edges.

3.5   Deep Belief Network Applications

Deep Belief Networks (DBNs) can be used frequently to create and recognize medical image, speech or sound signal processing, and predict differences. Some application examples of these studies are given below.

Liang et al. used DBN to analyze data in the Hospital Information System (HIS) and Electronic Medical Records (EMR). The application consists of two stages. In the first stage, features extraction was performed with DBN. In the second step, classification of these properties was done by conventional support vector machine. The results obtained from experimental studies show that the proposed mixed method provides much better performance than traditional methods [39].

Deep belief networks (DBNs) have examples of application for time series data to EEG analysis. DBNs were applied in a semi-controlled paradigm to model EEG waveforms for a classification and an abnormality detection. DBN performance was compared with standard classifiers for the same EEG dataset and the classification time was 1.7–103.7 times faster than other high-performance classifiers. From their results, they stated that raw data entries of DBNs may be more effective than other common techniques for online automatic EEG waveform recognition [40]. Freuden-burg et al. investigated the performance of DBNs to reduce the ECoG signal stream to several components that most directly correspond to the neural patterns associated with the task's performance (neural correlations) of the subject. They have developed a real-time feedback system based on real-time and incremental learning from DBN, which called "Brain Mirror". They showed that in the real patient data, the components learned online with DBN correlated with more neural patterns than PCA [41].

DBN is also widely used for the identification of such time series expansions with mixed methods using one or more stacked Restricted Boltzmann Machine (RBM). For examples, Al-Fatlawi et al. a DBN used the deep network formed by two stacked Restricted Boltzmann Machines (RBM) and an output layer to classify Parkinson's disease from speech signals. The learning phase in the network consists of two stages. In the first stage, it uses RBMs as unsupervised learning. In the second stage, they used the back-propagation algorithm as fine tuning. To demonstrate the effectiveness of the proposed system, experimental results have been compared with different approaches and related studies and are an effective method for diagnosing Parkinson's disease using the speech signal and DBN [42]. In a similar study, Taji et al. proposed an algorithm based on Deep Belief Networks (DBN), which can distinguish between noisy and clean signal measurements. The algorithm uses a three-layer stacked RBMs. The first two RBMs have been trained to classify and select data and apply them to the third layer of RBMs. Using the MIT-BIH Arrhythmia database, they found that the algorithm can successfully separate a noisy ECG signal from a clean signal [43]. In another study, An et al. proposed using the DBN, RBM, and Contrastive Divergence algorithms which aim to classify EEG data according to the Motor Imagery task. They compared the proposed method with support vector machines and found that deep learning was more effective [44].

In their study, Sun et al. Tested the efficiency of using deep learning algorithms for the diagnosis of lung cancer from Lung Images, and also compared the performance of deep learning algorithms. For this purpose, they used CTs in the Lung Image Database Consortium (LIDC) database and 3 separate deep networks such as Convolutional Neural Network (CNN), Deep Belief Networks (DBNs), Stacked Denoising Automatic Encoder (SDAE). The nodules on each computed tomography (CT) slice were segmented according to the signs provided by radiologists. They are categorized with 174,412 samples, each with 52×52 pixels and corresponding accuracy files. They used the support vector machine (SVM) with 28 image features to compare the performance of the deep learning algorithms. They found the accuracy of CNN, DBN and SDAE to be 0.7976, 0.8119 and 0.7929, and SVM 0.7940, respectively. The SVM classification accuracy rate was slightly lower than that of CNN and DBN. As seen in this example application, although there is not much DBN's for medical image processing in medical applications, DBNs give very good results in medical image processing. Even slightly, they perform better than CNN [45]. In another study by Sun et al., nodules were grouped according to the diagnosis of four radiologists. In this study, three deep learning methods were used: convolutional neural network (CNN), deep belief network (DBN) and stacked denoising autoencoder (SDAE). A system using hand-crafted features was used for comparative testing. According to the results obtained, the accuracy rate of the test system was found to be $0.848 \pm$

0.026 and the accuracy rate of CNN was 0.899 ± 0.018. DBN's accuracy rate was slightly higher in the test system, whereas SDAE was slightly lower [46].

Although DBN is used in general deep learning applications such as image processing, video motion recognition and speech recognition, it is generally used in medical applications for processing time series expansions. In other words, heart sounds are preferred for the analysis of EEG, ECG, and similar medical signals. In addition, although there is not much DBN's medical image processing in medical applications, DBNs give very good results in medical image processing. DBN could perform as well as CNN.

3.6 Deep Reinforcement Learning Applications

As a sub-branch of machine learning, reinforcement learning (RL) aims to strengthen the experience of interaction with the world and the behavioral decision-making capabilities using evaluative feedback. Unlike traditional supervised learning methods, which are often based on one-off, comprehensive and supervised reward signals, the RL solves problems related to simultaneously sampled, evaluative, and delayed feedback. Such distinguishing features make the RL technique a suitable candidate for developing powerful solutions in which the diagnosis of decisions or treatment regimens in various diagnostic areas is often characterized by a long and sequential procedure [47]. RL can be used in areas such as deriving dynamic information from biological data from multiple levels to reduce data redundancy, to discover new biomarkers for disease detection and prevention. However, there are some limitations and the need for improvements in the use of RL in bioinformatics. For example, unattended new learning is required for deep RL methods to reduce the need for large tagged data sets during the training phase. The multitasking and multivariate learning paradigm must progress to deal with dynamically changing problems [48]. Practices have been made in almost all areas of medical diagnosis with reinforcement learning. Some applications are given below.

Asoh et al. sought to obtain recommendations for Bayes inverse RL diabetes treatment from longitudinal medical records of diabetic patients. They stated that their results were promising [49]. Raghu used RL to learn effective medical treatment policies for sepsis, a dangerous health condition, from observational data. He compared the results of his application for the treatment of sepsis. He stated that Q-learning and Deep Q-Learning studies give the most effective results [50]. Liu et al. also proposed a two-stage method for predicting optimal Dynamic Therapy Regimens from observational medical data. Developed to provide data-driven personalized decision recommendations to physicians and patients, this method includes supervised learning to predict specialist actions in the first stage and DRL learning steps to predict the long-term value function of Dynamic Therapy Regimens. They tested the proposed method on a data set from the International Bone Marrow Transplant Research Center (CIBMTR) registration database, attempting to predict the order of prevention and treatment of acute and chronic grafts and host diseases after transplantation. It is stated that their predictions are very accurate [51].

Ling and his colleagues recommend an RL-containing approach to clinical diagnosis in their articles. They reported that during training, the RL agent mimicked the clinician's cognitive process and learned the most appropriate policy for obtaining the most appropriate diagnoses for a clinical narrative. Diagnostic estimates were obtained by analyzing the sentences in candidate diagnoses from external sources with RL in clinical context. A deep Q-network architecture is trained to optimize a reward function that measures the accuracy of candidate diagnoses. At the end of the experiments conducted on TREC CDS datasets, the proposed method was very effective [52]. Online symptom-checking sites are available, such as WebMD and Mayo Clinic, to identify possible causes and treatments for diseases based on a patient's symptoms. These sites attempt to predict a disease by asking a patient a series of questions about their symptoms and evaluating them. A symptom controller has two design objectives, such as ensuring high accuracy and intuitive interactions. In this context, Kao et al. have proposed context-sensitive hierarchical RL, which significantly increases the accuracy of symptom control on conventional systems and also conducts a limited number of investigations [53].

Netto and his colleagues have proposed an RL-containing method to solve the problem of classification of lung nodules in their articles. They used 3D geometric nodule properties to obtain properties in the classification. They stated that the obtained results were very encouraging, indicating that the RL classifier, which uses the characteristics of the geometry of the nodules, could effectively classify benign ones from malignant lung nodules than those using CT images. On the other hand, they emphasized that the learning phase takes a long time and the shortening of this process should be investigated [54]. Dai et al. proposed a method using RL to automatically track elongated structures such as axons and blood vessels, which is a difficult procedure in the field of biomedical imaging. In this method, they taught how to track a continuous action area by applying sub pixel level RL on simple synthetic data. They tested this network on two photon microscopy images. The proposed method gives better results than a standard analysis package for neuronal microscopy despite the field gap. They have shown better results when finely tuning real data or training with real tagged data [55]. Maicias et al. proposed a method based on RL to automatically detect the rate of breast lesions from contrast-enhanced magnetic resonance volumes (DCE-MRI). They used the screening tool, called the attention mechanism, to train a search policy to learn lesion detection and indicated that it accelerated the detection of lesions of very different structures. They tested this method by expanding the Q-network approach in a data set containing 117 DCE-MRI volumes to demonstrate lesion detection accuracy and acceleration [56]. In another study for image classification, Park et al. proposed a new method to train the reward-based active learning algorithm using reverse RL and the network of actor critics. This method of semi-supervised amplified active learning was tested on a U-Net segmentation network for pulmonary nodules on chest X-rays. The proposed method demonstrated the ability to effectively reduce the labeling load by achieving

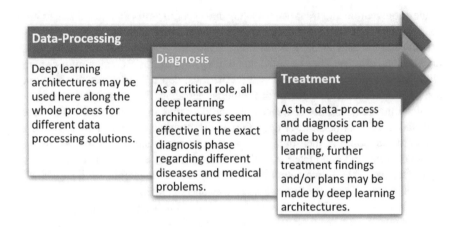

Fig. 3.2 Employment of deep learning architectures within medical and decision making

the same level of performance as the standard UNet while using only 50% of the tagged data [57].

As can be seen from the applications given above, deep reinforcement networks are often used to extract or estimate large and variable data such as clinical or health records. It is also often used for the classification and differentiation of very different medical images. Thus, it has emerged that RL can be used in many medical diagnosis and treatment fields.

As moving from the explanations so far, it is possible to draw a general mechanism of deep learning architectures for using towards decision support. By eliminating the details, a general flow regarding how different deep learning architectures can be employed in the context of medical applications can be drawn as in Fig. 3.2.

3.7   Applications with Other Deep Learning Architectures

In addition to the deep learning methods given above, there are many deep learning methods and applications that can be used as single or hybrid applications. Some applications are given below.

When we look at DBM applications, we see that it is generally used in image processing. For example, Cao et al. proposed a two-stage approach to medical imaging based on statistical graphical model and deep learning. First of all, they form the Secret Semantic Analysis model to obtain semantic data by taking visual and textual information from medical images. Then, they develop a DBM-based multimodal learning model to learn the common density model from multi-mode information to achieve missing modality. They have shown that the proposed method is very efficient for the medical imaging indexing and access system with applications made with a large number of medical images [58]. Wu et al. developed a shape model-oriented level determination method using DBM for heart movement monitoring. For the proposed method, they used a heart shape model that characterizes statistical variations in heart shapes in an exercise data set. This mechanism was created by training three-tier DBM to characterize both local and spherical heart shape variations. A cine MRI image sequence and a square image acquisition and testing system for the heart were established and tested using 38 coronal cine MRI image sequences. They stated that monitoring the heart movements of the system is very suitable for diagnosis [59].

As mentioned before, the Restricted Boltzmann Machine is also one of the deep learning methods that are widely used in medical applications. In his studies, Tomczak argued that RBM should be used as an independent nonlinear classifier that could be extremely useful in medical fields. In addition, it has shown how rare representation in RBM can be achieved by adding a regulatory term to the learning objective. He tested the method by applying it to five different medical fields [60, 61]. In their study, Zang et al. focused on the use of a two-stage DL to automatically extract image characteristics learned from shear wave elastography (SWE) data and to distinguish differences between benign and malignant breast tumors. In order to extract the SWE characteristics, they created a two-layer DL structure consisting of a Boltzmann machine with point gates (PGBM) and a restricted Boltzmann machine (RBM). The system consisted of SWE images of 22 ben, 135 benign tumors and 92 malignant tumors from 121 patients. It has been suggested that this method based on PGBM and RBM can be used in the computer aided clinical diagnosis of breast cancer from SWE images [62]. RBM has also been applied for the diagnosis of breast cancer by classifying images. Histopathological breast-cancer images were used in the application. The Histopathological breast-cancer images were obtained from the BreakHis dataset [63].

Tran et al. proposed a method for utilizing electronic medical record (EMR) using RBM with minimal human intervention. This method, which they call EMR-driven non-negative RBM, derives a new representation of medical objects by placing them in a low-dimensional vector space. They tested the ability of ENRBM on a cohort of 7578 mental health patients under suicide risk assessment. It was stated that the results obtained were significantly higher than those obtained from clinicians and those obtained with support vector machines [64].

Stacked autoencoder neural network (SAE) is one of the most frequently used methods in medical diagnosis. Kannadasan et al. using the features of Pima Indian diabetes data, they have detected Type 2 diabetes with stacked auto-encoders. They stated that the proposed method showed a high success rate with 86.26% accuracy rate [65]. Zang et al. proposed a stacked denoising auto-encoder neural network (SDAE) algorithm based on cost-sensitive over-sampling in order to solve the over-fitting and noise problems of the over-sampling algorithm when synthesizing new minority class samples of a network. They stated that the proposed algorithm showed that unbalanced datasets improved the classification accuracy of the minority class [66]. In another medical database diagnostic application, Kadam et al. to classify breast cancer as non-cancerous and cancerous, they suggested learning a group of features based on the Stacked Sparse Autoencoders (SSAE) and Softmax Regression.

In practice, they used the Wisconsin Breast Cancer data set from the UCI machine learning database. A high accuracy of classification had achieved with 98.60% [67]. Sadati et al. in their study, they proposed an approach based on feature representations and word placement techniques using DL methods. In the method, they used 4 different DL techniques: stacked sparse autoencoders, deep belief network, adversarial autoencoders and variational autoencoders to obtain effective and robust features from EHRs. They emphasized that the proposed method is more suitable for datasets with little or no tagged data. As a result of the application, they stated that stacked sparse autoencoders showed superior overall performance for small data sets and variational autoencoders performed better than other techniques for large data sets [68].

Jia et al. in their study, they developed a pathological brain detection system to classify pathological brain images into five healthy categories such as cerebrovascular disease, neoplastic disease, degenerative disease, and inflammatory disease. In the proposed method, they used a softmax layer for grading with a deep-stacked sparse autoencoder. As a result, the accuracy of the deep-stacked sparse autoencoder on the test set was found to be 98.6%. Estimation time of each image in the test phase was found to be only 0.070 s. It shows that SSAE is able to classify very quickly [69]. Shin et al. used 4D patient data and multi-organ detection by performing unchecked feature learning in stacked autoencoders. In other words, deep learning methods were applied to make multi-organ identification in the MRI medical images. They extracted visual and temporal hierarchical features that learned to classify object classes from an unlabeled multimode DCE-MRI dataset for classifiers. They used a probabilistic patch-based method for the detection of multiple organs with features learned by SAE. They have demonstrated that the proposed method can be used efficiently in unlabeled datasets or a missing data in datasets [70]. A feature extraction method for medical images with DL has also been proposed by Sharma and colleagues. They used SAE, which encoded images into binary vectors. To test the performance of the proposed method, they used IRMA dataset with 14,410 X-ray images. For this dataset, it was reported that SAE achieved excellent results with 37.6 retrieval errors for 1733 test images with 74.61% compression [71].

For data that is infrequently represented in the CNN, there may be representative loss. In RNN, gradient losses in weak input sequences may occur. These types of CNN and RNN are used in conjunction with techniques such as long short-term memory unit (LSTM) and Gated recurrent units (GRUs) to eliminate some representation constraints. Long short term memory units (LSTMs) or Gated recurrent units (GRUs) are used to briefly use sequential information of input data by cyclic connections between respective units such as sensors. Some applications of these are given below.

Kim et al. have focused on estimating missing examination data in EHR, addressing the problems that electronic health records will cause in a future machine learning. For this purpose, they tried to estimate the missing data by using RNN and LSTM. They tested the proposed method using the Korean people's medical examination database. In this database, they conducted all medical studies in 13 clinics for 12 consecutive years. Every year, 11,500 people had medical examinations and 7400 people missed interim examinations. They tried to estimate the data that may be present in these missing examinations by training the proposed model with complete data first. According to the results obtained, the proposed method predicts much better than traditional linear regression in most of the examination [72]. Lipton et al. conducted another medical diagnostic application with RNN and LSTM for irregular sequences data in EHRs. They stated that medical data, especially in units such as emergency services, can be thought of as time series for each stage is recorded in EHRs. However, many EHR recordings may have deficiencies or have very variable data. They selected RNN and LSTM hybrid methods as the DL method to make an appropriate diagnosis from the data group consisting of these irregular sequences. In particular, considering the multi-label classification of diagnoses, they have developed a model to classify 128 diagnoses in 13 clinics for frequently given but irregularly sampled clinical measurements. They suggest that the proposed method performs better than many powerful estimation methods [73].

We can give an example for a hybrid DL method which include a RNN using GRU. Choi and colleagues tried to predict the initial diagnosis of heart failure with RNN using GRU to model the temporal relationships between events in EHRs. For this purpose, they used a data group with 3884 heart failure in a total of 28,903 health controls. They have developed a model to determine the relationships between cases, such as disease diagnosis, drug orders, and procedural orders, over a 12–18-month case and control observation interval. They compared the criteria with regular logistic regression, neural network, support vector machine and K-nearest neighbor classifier approaches to test the performance of the proposed model. The accuracy of the classifiers for the 12-month baseline range is 0.777 for RNN, 0.747 for logistic regression, 0.765 for multi-layer sensor (MLP), 0.743 for support vector machine (SVM), and 0.730 for K-nearest neighbor (KNN). The accuracy of the classifiers for the 18-month basic interval is 0.883 for RNN and 0.834 for MLP, respectively. From these results, it is seen that RNN using GRU for the diagnosis of heart failure based on time from EHR provides the highest accuracy rates [74].

A CNN and a LSTM are widely used together to predict a medical diagnosis from medical dataset or medical images. In their study, Rahman and Adjeroh attempted to estimate the biological age of adult humans CNN and LSTM from these data by recording human physical activities using a wearable device. They used the NHANES physical activity data set, which included five sets of deep biological age estimates, to test the proposed method. According to their results, the proposed method performs better than other state-of-the-art approaches for biological age estimation [75]. Ordóñez and Roggen, also used CNN and LSTM to differentiate the activities of adult people by recording human physical activities with the help of a wearable device and explained the advantages of the proposed method [76]. Here, it can be said that CNN and LSTM hybrid method is firstly preferred and efficient results are obtained for the classification of raw data from sensors to detect such mobile activities.

CNN and LSTM are used for image processing. Aditi et al. they attempted to diagnose breast cancer using the LSTM-CNN layered structure. Invasive ductal carcinoma (IDC) created by Cruz-Roa et al. Used all slide images (WSI) to test their proposed method. They first classified the dataset separately with CNN and LSTM, and then combined LSTM-CNN together. LSTM-CNN obtained the highest accuracy rate of the classification accuracy obtained. In the separate study, the accuracy rate obtained by LSTM was higher than that of CNN. Thus, as mentioned earlier, the performance of the mixed methods is often higher than the single use of DLs [77].

To support medical diagnosis, reliable sources such as medical images, laboratory test results are used. The fact that these methods are too large and often patient-specific (unique) makes it difficult for both health care workers and clinical support systems using DL to obtain clear information. There are also limitations in DL applications. For example, it is very difficult for a network to be trained for majority data to generalize and obtain information from minority representations in a given scenario. Likewise, if a controlled learning method is used, it is very difficult to obtain a fully labeled series of training data from complex medical images or non-linear medical data of different sizes. When analyzing new minority class samples of medical data, problems arise with over-fitting and noise problems of the model, which makes it difficult to obtain accurate information. To overcome these problems, the use of hybrid DL techniques in medical diagnostic DL applications has increased.

Researchers have put forward many different models and their reasons for analyzing the missing and different medical data and obtaining the correct information. Both CNNs and LSTM have shown improvements in DNNs in a wide variety of speech recognition tasks. For example, Sainath et al. in their study, CNNs, LSTMs and DNNs are complementary to the modeling capabilities because CNNs are good at reducing frequency variations, LSTMs are good at transient modeling, and DNNs are suitable to map properties to a more distinct area [78]. Although it is not seen in practice, there is a possibility to use medical diagnosis of Parkinson's and Alzheimer's diseases from speech records and to obtain effective diagnosis.

As can be seen from the applications listed above, if we list the hybrid methods used for modeling and providing a good generalization of the underrepresented data by making a good feature extraction from the missing, complex, irregular and more importantly unlabeled data; CNN-LSTM, RNN-LSTM, and DBN-RBM are generally used for medical image processing. Enhanced autoencoder types, such as SAE, SDAE or SSAE, are often used to process both irregular medical data and medical images. Further, autoencoder-CNN or RNN-CNN hybrid methods are available as shown in some applications above.

Considering the explained state of the literature of deep learning for medical problems (especially diagnosis/decision support), it can be seen that some architectures may be seen more used rather than the other ones. As that situation may change in time, it is possible to give a general usage ranking of the related architectures as in Fig. 3.3.

3.8   Summary

As the most widely used architecture, there are many studies conducted with CNN for different diseases that cannot be mentioned here. Here in this chapter, just a few

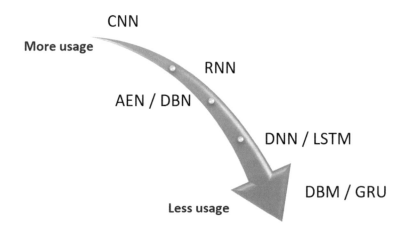

Fig. 3.3 General usage ranking of the deep learning architectures in terms of medical problems

application examples are expressed as the research in recent years for different topics. As can be seen from the given applications, CNNs are often used for the processing and classification of medical images. In other words, CNNs or hybrid CNNs are the first solutions that come to mind for a computer-assisted diagnostic system to be created by evaluating medical images.

Just as in CNNs, many more medical diagnoses application examples can be given for RNNs. As can be seen from the applications given, RNNs are generally one of the most preferred methods for time series solutions. In this context, it is used for the processing and classification of all medical signals that can be considered as natural language analysis or time series expansion. In other words, RNNs or hybrid RNNs are the first solutions that come to mind for a computer-assisted diagnostic system to obtain an optimal prediction by evaluating medical signals (such as ECG, PCG, EEG) or data that may vary greatly over time (i.e. EHR).

AENs are generally one of the most preferred methods for large numerical data or statistical analysis. In this context, it is used for the processing and classification of all medical signals or medical data, which can be obtained with equal weighted features (i.e. features vectors or matrices). In other words, AENs or hybrid AENs are the first solutions that come to mind for a computer-assisted diagnostic system to be created by evaluating medical signals (such as ECG, PCG, EEG) or very large data.

Although DNNs are generally one of the preferred methods for very large complex medical data or statistical analysis, they can be used in medical image processing and a segmentation of medical images or a selection of image edges.

Although DBN is used in general deep learning applications such as image processing, video motion recognition and speech recognition, it is generally used in medical applications for processing time series expansions. In other words, heart sounds are preferred for the analysis of EEG, ECG, and similar medical signals. In addition, although there is not much medical image processing in DBN medical applications, DBNs give very good results in medical image processing. DBN perform as well as CNN.

Also, deep reinforcement networks are often used to extract or estimate large and variable data such as clinical or health records. It is also often used for the classification and differentiation of very different medical images. Thus, it has emerged that RL can be used in many medical diagnosis and treatment fields.

For data that is infrequently represented in the CNN, there may be representative loss. In RNN, gradient losses in weak input sequences may occur. These types of CNN and RNN are used in conjunction with techniques such as long short-term memory unit (LSTM) and gated recurrent units (GRUs) to eliminate some representation constraints. Long short term memory units (LSTMs) or gated recurrent units (GRUs) are used to briefly use sequential information of input data by cyclic connections between respective units such as sensors.

We see that Deep Boltzmann Machine (DBM) is generally used in image processing. The Restricted Boltzmann Machine (RBM) is also one of the deep learning methods that are widely used in medical applications. RBM should be used as an independent nonlinear classifier that could be extremely useful in medical fields.

For data that is infrequently represented in the CNN, there may be representative loss. In RNN, gradient losses in weak input sequences may occur. These types of CNN and RNN are used in conjunction with techniques such as long short-term memory unit (LSTM) and gated recurrent units (GRUs) to eliminate some representation constraints. Long short term memory units (LSTMs) or gated recurrent units (GRUs) are used to briefly use sequential information of input data by cyclic connections between respective units such as sensors. Some examples of these are given below.

To support medical diagnosis, reliable sources such as medical images, laboratory test results are used. The fact that these methods are too large and often patient-specific (unique) makes it difficult for both health care workers and clinical support systems using DL to obtain clear information. There are also limitations in DL applications. For example, it is very difficult for a network to be trained for majority data to generalize and obtain information from minority representations in a given scenario. Likewise, if a controlled learning method is used, it is very difficult to obtain a fully labeled series of training data from complex medical images or non-linear medical data of different sizes. When analyzing new minority class samples of medical data, problems arise with over-fitting and noise problems of the model, which makes it difficult to obtain accurate information. To overcome these problems, the use of hybrid DL techniques in medical diagnostic DL applications has increased.

Hybrid methods used to model and provide a good generalization of inadequately represented data by extracting good property from missing, complex, irregular and more importantly unlabeled data can be listed as follows. CNN-LSTM and RNN-LSTM are often used for medical image processing. Advanced autoencoder types such as SAE, SDAE or SSAE are often used to process both non-regular medical data and medical images. In addition, autoencoder-CNN or RNN-CNN hybrid methods are also used.

After understanding more about essentials of different deep learning architectures and their applications in the context of medical applications (considering decision support potentials), some of recent research ways can be explained in detail. The next chapters are devoted to some of remarkable diagnosis efforts for specific diseases.

3.9 Further Learning

In order to have more idea about how traditional machine learning and general artificial intelligence algorithms—techniques were used for medical diagnosis problems, readers can read [79–87].

As deep learning has also many more examples of applications in cancer-oriented research, the readers can read some very recent ones from [88–92].

Since it is important that hybrid systems can improve research findings in terms of medical diagnosis, some recent examples can be read from [93–100].

Also, some of the recent books to read about machine learning—deep learning perspectives in healthcare, medical diagnosis and other related subjects are [101–104].

References

1. M. Bakator, D. Radosav, Deep learning and medical diagnosis: a review of literature. Multimodal Technol. Interact. **2**(3), 47 (2018)
2. R. Neelapu, G.L. Devi, K.S. Rao, Deep learning based conventional neural network architecture for medical image classification. Traitement du Signal **35**(2), 169 (2018)
3. O. Deperlioglu, Classification of phonocardiograms with convolutional neural networks. BRAIN. Broad Res. Artif. Intell. Neurosci. **9**(2), 22–33 (2018)
4. O. Deperlioglu, Classification of segmented phonocardiograms by convolutional neural networks. BRAIN. Broad Res. Artif. Intell. Neurosci. **10**(2), 5–13 (2019)
5. H. Fujita, D. Cimr, Computer aided detection for fibrillations and flutters using deep convolutional neural network. Inf. Sci. **486**, 231–239 (2019)
6. D.J. Hemanth, O. Deperlioglu, U. Kose, An enhanced diabetic retinopathy detection and classification approach using deep convolutional neural network. Neural Comput. Appl. 1–15 (2020)
7. O. Deperlıoğlu, U. Kose, Diagnosis of diabetic retinopathy by using image processing and convolutional neural network, in *2018 2nd International Symposium on Multidisciplinary Studies and Innovative Technologies (ISMSIT)* (IEEE, 2018), pp. 1–5
8. L.C. Afonso, G.H. Rosa, C.R. Pereira, S.A. Weber, C. Hook, V.H.C. Albuquerque, J.P. Papa, A recurrence plot-based approach for Parkinson's disease identification. Fut. Gener. Comput. Syst. **94**, 282–292 (2019)
9. M. Längkvist, J. Jendeberg, P. Thunberg, A. Loutfi, M. Lidén, Computer aided detection of ureteral stones in thin slice computed tomography volumes using Convolutional Neural Networks. Comput. Biol. Med. **97**, 153–160 (2018)
10. S. Iqbal, M.U. Ghani, T. Saba, A. Rehman, Brain tumor segmentation in multi-spectral MRI using convolutional neural networks (CNN). Microsc. Res. Tech. **81**(4), 419–427 (2018)

11. Z. Yan, Y. Zhan, Z. Peng, S. Liao, Y.. Shinagawa, S. Zhang, X.S. Zhou, Multi-instance deep learning: discover discriminative local anatomies for bodypart recognition. IEEE Trans. Med. Imaging **35**(5), 1332–1343 (2016)
12. Y. Bar, I. Diamant, L. Wolf, H. Greenspan, Deep learning with non-medical training used for chest pathology identification, in *Medical Imaging 2015: Computer-Aided Diagnosis*, vol. 9414 (International Society for Optics and Photonics, 2015), pp. 94140V, Mar 2015
13. S. Okamoto, T. Yokota, J.H. Lee, A. Takai, T. Kido, M. Matsuda, *Detection of Hepatocellular Carcinoma in CT Images Using Deep Learning* (2018)
14. J. Cho, K. Lee, E. Shin, G. Choy, & S. Do, Medical image deep learning with hospital PACS dataset (2015). arXiv preprint arXiv:1511.06348
15. S. Min, B. Lee, S. Yoon, Deep learning in bioinformatics. Brief. Bioinform. **18**(5), 851–869 (2017)
16. S. Tanwar, J. Jotheeswaran, Survey on deep learning for medical imaging. JASC J. Appl. Sci. Comput. **5**(7), 1608–1620 (2018)
17. N.F. Güler, E.D. Übeyli, I. Güler, Recurrent neural networks employing Lyapunov exponents for EEG signals classification. Expert Syst. Appl. **29**(3), 506–514 (2005)
18. E.D. Übeyli, Implementing automated diagnostic systems for breast cancer detection. Expert Syst. Appl. **33**(4), 1054–1062 (2007)
19. H. Al-Askar, N. Radi, Á. MacDermott, Recurrent neural networks in medical data analysis and classifications, in *Applied Computing in Medicine and Health* (Morgan Kaufmann, 2016), pp. 147–165
20. Y. Mu, M. Huang, C. Ye, Q. Wu, Diagnosis prediction via recurrent neural networks. Int. J. Mach. Learn. Comput. **8**(2) (2018)
21. E. Choi, M.T. Bahadori, A. Schuetz, W.F. Stewart, J. Sun, Doctor ai: Predicting clinical events via recurrent neural networks, in *Machine Learning for Healthcare Conference* (2016, December), pp. 301–318
22. A.N. Jagannatha, H. Yu, Bidirectional RNN for medical event detection in electronic health records, in *Proceedings of the Conference. Association for Computational Linguistics. North American Chapter. Meeting*, vol. 2016. NIH Public Access (2016, June), p. 473
23. M. Seera, C.P. Lim, K.S. Tan, W.S. Liew, Classification of transcranial Doppler signals using individual and ensemble recurrent neural networks. Neurocomputing **249**, 337–344 (2017)
24. J. Szkoła, K. Pancerz, J. Warchoł, Recurrent neural networks in computer-based clinical decision support for laryngopathies: an experimental study. Comput. Intell. Neurosci. **2011**, 7 (2011)
25. O. Deperlioglu, Classification of segmented heart sounds with autoencoder neural networks, in *VIII. International Multidisciplinary Congress of Eurasia* (IMCOFE'2019). ISBN: 978–605-68882-6-7, pp. 122-128, 24–26 Apr 2019, Antalya
26. O. Deperlioğlu, The effects of different training algorithms on the classification of medical databases using artificial neural networks, in *2nd European Conference on Science, Art & Culture (ECSAC 2018)*, Antalya, Turkey between April 19 to 22, 2018. ISBN: 978-605-288-553-6, pp. 91–98
27. O. Deperlioglu, Hepatitis disease diagnosis with deep neural networks, in *International 4th European Conference on Science, Art & Culture (ECSAC'2019)*. ISBN: 978-605-7809-73-5, pp. 467–473, 18 to 21 Apr 2019, Antalya
28. O. Deperlioglu, Using autoencoder deep neural networks for diagnosis of breast cancer, in *International 4th European Conference on Science, Art & Culture (ECSAC'2019)*, ISBN: 978-605-7809-73-5, pp. 475-481, 18 to 21 Apr 2019, Antalya
29. D. Arifoglu, A. Bouchachia, Activity recognition and abnormal behaviour detection with recurrent neural networks. Procedia Comput. Sci. **110**, 86–93 (2017)
30. K. Mao, R. Tang, X. Wang, W. Zhang, H. Wu, Feature representation using deep autoencoder for lung nodule image classification. *Complexity* (2018)
31. M. Chen, X. Shi, Y. Zhang, D. Wu, M. Guizani, Deep features learning for medical image analysis with convolutional autoencoder neural network. IEEE Trans. Big Data (2017)

32. M.S. Ayhan, L. Kuehlewein, G. Aliyeva, W. Inhoffen, F. Ziemssen, P. Berens, Expert-validated estimation of diagnostic uncertainty for deep neural networks in diabetic retinopathy detection. *medRxiv*, 19002154 (2019)

33. C. Leibig, V. Allken, M.S. Ayhan et al., Leveraging uncertainty information from deep neural networks for disease detection. Sci. Rep. **7**, 17816 (2017). https://doi.org/10.1038/s41598-017-17876-z

34. Q. Li, B. Feng, L. Xie, P. Liang, H. Zhang, T. Wang, A cross-modality learning approach for vessel segmentation in retinal images. IEEE Trans. Med. Imaging **35**(1), 109–118 (2015)

35. K.H. Miaoa, J.H. Miaoa, Coronary Heart Disease Diagnosis using Deep Neural Networks. Int. J. Adv. Comput. Sci. Appl. **9**(10), 1–8 (2018)

36. R.R. Agravat, & M.S. Raval, Deep learning for automated brain tumor segmentation in MRI Images, in *Soft Computing Based Medical Image Analysis* (pp. 183–201). Academic Press (2018)

37. D.C. Cireşan, A. Giusti, L.M. Gambardella, J. Schmidhuber, Mitosis detection in breast cancer histology images with deep neural networks, in *International Conference on Medical Image Computing and Computer-assisted Intervention* (Springer, Berlin, 2013), Sept 2013, pp. 411–418

38. R. Shimizu, S. Yanagawa, Y. Monde, H. Yamagishi, M. Hamada, T. Shimizu, T. Kuroda, Deep learning application trial to lung cancer diagnosis for medical sensor systems, in *2016 International SoC Design Conference (ISOCC)* (IEEE, 2016), Oct 2016, pp. 191–192

39. Z. Liang, G. Zhang, J.X. Huang, Q.V.Hu, Deep learning for healthcare decision making with EMRs, in *2014 IEEE International Conference on Bioinformatics and Biomedicine (BIBM)*. IEEE (2014, November), pp. 556–559

40. D.F. Wulsin, J.R. Gupta, R. Mani, J.A. Blanco, B. Litt, Modeling electroencephalography waveforms with semi-supervised deep belief nets: fast classification and anomaly measurement. J. Neural Eng. **8**(3), 036015 (2011)

41. Z.V. Freudenburg, N.F. Ramsey, M. Wronkiewicz, W.D. Smart, R. Pless, E.C. Leuthardt, Real-time naive learning of neural correlates in ECoG electrophysiology. Int. J. Mach. Learn. Comput. **1**(3), 269 (2011)

42. A.H. Al-Fatlawi, M.H. Jabardi, S.H. Ling, Efficient diagnosis system for Parkinson's disease using deep belief network, in *2016 IEEE Congress on Evolutionary Computation (CEC)*. IEEE (2016, July), pp. 1324–1330

43. B. Taji, A.D. Chan, S. Shirmohammadi, Classifying measured electrocardiogram signal quality using deep belief networks, in *2017 IEEE International Instrumentation and Measurement Technology Conference (I2MTC)*. IEEE (2017, May), pp. 1–6

44. X. An, D. Kuang, X. Guo, Y. Zhao, L. He, A deep learning method for classification of EEG data based on motor imagery, in *International Conference on Intelligent Computing*. Springer, Cham (2014, August), pp. 203–210

45. W. Sun, B. Zheng, W. Qian, Computer aided lung cancer diagnosis with deep learning algorithms, in *Medical imaging 2016: computer-aided diagnosis*, vol. 9785 (International Society for Optics and Photonics, 2016, March), p. 97850Z

46. W. Sun, B. Zheng, W. Qian, Automatic feature learning using multichannel ROI based on deep structured algorithms for computerized lung cancer diagnosis. Comput. Biol. Med. **89**, 530–539 (2017)

47. C. Yu, J. Liu, S. Nemati, Reinforcement learning in healthcare: a survey (2019). arXiv preprint arXiv:1908.08796

48. M. Mahmud, M.S. Kaiser, A. Hussain, S. Vassanelli, Applications of deep learning and reinforcement learning to biological data. IEEE Transact. Neural Netw. Learn. Syst. **29**(6), 2063–2079 (2018)

49. H. Asoh, M.S.S. Akaho, T. Kamishima, K. Hasida, E. Aramaki, T. Kohro, An application of inverse reinforcement learning to medical records of diabetes treatment, in *ECMLPKDD2013 Workshop on Reinforcement Learning with Generalized Feedback* (2013, September)

50. A. Raghu, Reinforcement learning for sepsis treatment: baselines and analysis, in *ICML 2019 Workshop* (2019)

51. N. Liu, Y. Liu, B. Logan, Z. Xu, J. Tang, Y. Wang, Learning the dynamic treatment regimes from medical registry data through deep Q-network. Sci. Rep. **9**(1), 1495 (2019)
52. Y. Ling, S.A. Hasan, V. Datla, A. Qadir, K. Lee, J. Liu, O. Farri, Learning to diagnose: assimilating clinical narratives using deep reinforcement learning, in *Proceedings of the Eighth International Joint Conference on Natural Language Processing (Volume 1: Long Papers)* (pp. 895–905) (2017, November)
53. H.C. Kao, K.F. Tang, E.Y. Chang, Context-aware symptom checking for disease diagnosis using hierarchical reinforcement learning, in *Thirty-Second AAAI Conference on Artificial Intelligence* (2018, April)
54. S.M.B. Netto, V.R.C. Leite, A.C. Silva, A.C. de Paiva,, A. de Almeida Neto, Application on reinforcement learning for diagnosis based on medical image. *Reinforcement Learning*, 379 (2008)
55. T. Dai, M. Dubois, K. Arulkumaran, J. Campbell, C. Bass, B. Billot, A.A. Bharath, et al., Deep reinforcement learning for subpixel neural tracking, in *International Conference on Medical Imaging with Deep Learning* (2019, May), pp. 130–150
56. G. Maicas, G. Carneiro, A.P. Bradley, J.C. Nascimento, I. Reid, Deep reinforcement learning for active breast lesion detection from DCE-MRI, in *International Conference on Medical Image Computing and Computer-Assisted Intervention*. Springer, Cham (2017, September), pp. 665–673
57. S. Park, W. Hwang, K.H. Jung, Semi-supervised reinforced active learning for pulmonary nodule detection in chest X-rays, in *Medical Imaging with Deep Learning, MIDL* (2018)
58. Y. Cao, S. Steffey, J. He, D. Xiao, C. Tao, P. Chen, H. Müller, Medical image retrieval: a multimodal approach. Cancer Inf. **13**, CIN-S14053 (2014)
59. J. Wu, T.R. Mazur, S. Ruan, C. Lian, N. Daniel, H. Lashmett, S. Mutic, A deep Boltzmann machine-driven level set method for heart motion tracking using cine MRI images. Med. Image Anal. **47**, 68–80 (2018)
60. J.M. Tomczak, Application of classification restricted Boltzmann machine to medical domains. World Appl. Sci. J. **31**, 69–75 (2014)
61. J.M. Tomczak, *Application of Classification Restricted Boltzmann Machine with discriminative and sparse learning to medical domains*. Institute of Computer Science Wroclaw University of Technology (2014)
62. Q. Zhang, Y. Xiao, W. Dai, J. Suo, C. Wang, J. Shi, H. Zheng, Deep learning based classification of breast tumors with shear-wave elastography. Ultrasonics **72**, 150–157 (2016)
63. A.A. Nahid, A. Mikaelian, Y. Kong, Histopathological breast-image classification with restricted Boltzmann machine along with backpropagation. Biomed. Res. **29**(10), 2068–2077 (2018)
64. T. Tran, T.D. Nguyen, D. Phung, S. Venkatesh, Learning vector representation of medical objects via EMR-driven nonnegative restricted Boltzmann machines (eNRBM). J. Biomed. Inform. **54**, 96–105 (2015)
65. K. Kannadasan, D.R. Edla, V. Kuppili, Type 2 diabetes data classification using stacked autoencoders in deep neural networks. Clin. Epidemiol. Global Health (2018). https://doi.org/10.1016/j.cegh.2018.12.004
66. C. Zhang, W. Gao, J. Song, J. Jiang, An imbalanced data classification algorithm of improved autoencoder neural network, in *2016 Eighth International Conference on Advanced Computational Intelligence (ICACI)*. IEEE (2016, February), pp. 95–99
67. V.J. Kadam, S.M. Jadhav, K. Vijayakumar, Breast cancer diagnosis using feature ensemble learning based on stacked sparse autoencoders and softmax regression. J. Med. Syst. **43**(8), 263 (2019)
68. N. Sadati, M.Z. Nezhad, R.B. Chinnam, D. Zhu, Representation learning with autoencoders for electronic health records: a comparative study (2019). arXiv preprint arXiv:1908.09174
69. W. Jia, K. Muhammad, S.H. Wang, Y.D. Zhang, Five-category classification of pathological brain images based on deep stacked sparse autoencoder. Multimedia Tools Appl. **78**(4), 4045–4064 (2019)

70. H.C. Shin, M.R. Orton, D.J. Collins, S.J. Doran, M.O. Leach, Stacked autoencoders for unsupervised feature learning and multiple organ detection in a pilot study using 4D patient data. IEEE Trans. Pattern Anal. Mach. Intell. **35**(8), 1930–1943 (2012)
71. S. Sharma, I. Umar, L. Ospina, D. Wong, H.R. Tizhoosh, Stacked autoencoders for medical image search, in *International Symposium on Visual Computing*. Springer, Cham (2016, December), pp. 45–54
72. H.G. Kim, G.J. Jang, H.J Choi, M. Kim, Y.W. Kim, J. Choi, Recurrent neural networks with missing information imputation for medical examination data prediction, in *2017 IEEE International Conference on Big Data and Smart Computing (BigComp)*. (IEEE, 2017, February), pp. 317–323
73. Z.C. Lipton, D.C. Kale, C. Elkan, R. Wetzel, Learning to diagnose with LSTM recurrent neural networks (2015). arXiv preprint arXiv:1511.03677
74. E. Choi, A. Schuetz, W.F. Stewart, J. Sun, Using recurrent neural network models for early detection of heart failure onset. J. Am. Med. Inform. Assoc. **24**(2), 361–370 (2016)
75. S.A. Rahman, D.A. Adjeroh, Deep Learning using Convolutional LSTM estimates Biological Age from Physical Activity. Sci. Rep. **9**(1), 1–15 (2019)
76. Ordóñez, F., D. Roggen, Deep convolutional and LSTM recurrent neural networks for multimodal wearable activity recognition. Sensors **16**(1), 115 (2016)
77. Aditi, M.K. Nagda, E. Poovammal, Image classification using a hybrid LSTM-CNN deep neural network. Int. J. Eng. Adv. Technol. (IJEAT), **8**(6), 1342–1348 (2019)
78. T.N. Sainath, O. Vinyals, A. Senior, H. Sak, Convolutional, long short-term memory, fully connected deep neural networks, in *2015 IEEE International Conference on Acoustics, Speech and Signal Processing (ICASSP)*. IEEE (2015, April), pp. 4580–4584
79. S.K. De, R. Biswas, A.R. Roy, An application of intuitionistic fuzzy sets in medical diagnosis. Fuzzy Sets Syst. **117**(2), 209–213 (2001)
80. F. Amato, A. López, E.M. Peña-Méndez, P. Vaňhara, A. Hampl, J. Havel, Artificial neural networks in medical diagnosis (2013)
81. K.P. Adlassnig, Fuzzy set theory in medical diagnosis. IEEE Trans. Syst. Man Cybernetics. **16**(2), 260–265 (1986)
82. I. Kononenko, Machine learning for medical diagnosis: history, state of the art and perspective. Artif. Intell. Med. **23**(1), 89–109 (2001)
83. I. Kononenko, Inductive and Bayesian learning in medical diagnosis. Appl. Artif. Intell. Int. J. **7**(4), 317–337 (1993)
84. J. Soni, U. Ansari, D. Sharma, S. Soni, Predictive data mining for medical diagnosis: an overview of heart disease prediction. Int. J. Comput. Appl. **17**(8), 43–48 (2011)
85. S. Ghumbre, C. Patil, A. Ghatol, Heart disease diagnosis using support vector machine, in *International Conference on Computer Science and Information Technology (ICCSIT') Pattaya* (2011)
86. N. Barakat, A.P. Bradley, M.N.H. Barakat, Intelligible support vector machines for diagnosis of diabetes mellitus. IEEE Trans. Inf Technol. Biomed. **14**(4), 1114–1120 (2010)
87. A.T. Azar, S.M. El-Metwally, Decision tree classifiers for automated medical diagnosis. Neural Comput. Appl. **23**(7–8), 2387–2403 (2013)
88. A. Yala, C. Lehman, T. Schuster, T. Portnoi, R. Barzilay, A deep learning mammography-based model for improved breast cancer risk prediction. Radiology **292**(1), 60–66 (2019)
89. J.N. Kather, A.T. Pearson, N. Halama, D. Jäger, J. Krause, S.H. Loosen, H.I. Grabsch, et al., Deep learning can predict microsatellite instability directly from histology in gastrointestinal cancer. Nat. Med. **25**(7), 1054–1056 (2019)
90. S.K. Lakshmanaprabu, S.N. Mohanty, K. Shankar, N. Arunkumar, G. Ramirez, Optimal deep learning model for classification of lung cancer on CT images. Fut. Gener. Comput. Syst. **92**, 374–382 (2019)
91. S. Khan, N. Islam, Z. Jan, I.U. Din, J.J.C. Rodrigues, A novel deep learning based framework for the detection and classification of breast cancer using transfer learning. Pattern Recogn. Lett. **125**, 1–6 (2019)

92. K. Nagpal, D. Foote, Y. Liu, P.H.C. Chen, E. Wulczyn, F. Tan, G.S. Corrado, et al. Development and validation of a deep learning algorithm for improving Gleason scoring of prostate cancer. NPJ Dig. Med. **2**(1), 1–10 (2019)
93. R. Yan, F. Ren, X. Rao, B. Shi, T. Xiang, L. Zhang, F. Zhang, et al., Integration of multimodal data for breast cancer classification using a hybrid deep learning method, in *International Conference on Intelligent Computing*. (Springer, Cham, 2019, August), pp. 460–469
94. K. Gjertsson, K. Johnsson, J. Richter, K. Sjöstrand, L. Edenbrandt, A. Anand, A novel automated deep learning algorithm for segmentation of the skeleton in low-dose CT for [(18) F] DCFPyL PET/CT hybrid imaging in patients with metastatic prostate cancer (2019)
95. H. Polat, H. Danaei Mehr, Classification of pulmonary CT images by using hybrid 3D-deep convolutional neural network architecture. Appl. Sci. **9**(5), 940 (2019)
96. L.J. Vaickus, A.A. Suriawinata, J.W. Wei, X. Liu, Automating the Paris System for urine cytopathology—a hybrid deep-learning and morphometric approach. Cancer Cytopathol. **127**(2), 98–115 (2019)
97. J. Van, C. Yoon, J. Glavis-Bloom, M. Bardis, A. Ushinsky, D.S. Chow, D. Fujimoto, et al., Deep learning hybrid 3D/2D convolutional neural network for prostate MRI recognition (2019)
98. S. Seth, B. Agarwal, A hybrid deep learning model for detecting diabetic retinopathy. J. Stat. Manag. Syst. **21**(4), 569–574 (2018)
99. G. Amit, O. Hadad, S. Alpert, T. Tlusty, Y. Gur, R. Ben-Ari, S. Hashoul, Hybrid mass detection in breast MRI combining unsupervised saliency analysis and deep learning, in *International Conference on Medical Image Computing and Computer-Assisted Intervention* (Springer, Cham, 2017), pp. 594–602
100. D. Maji, A. Santara, S. Ghosh, D. Sheet, P. Mitra, Deep neural network and random forest hybrid architecture for learning to detect retinal vessels in fundus images, in *2015 37th annual international conference of the IEEE Engineering in Medicine and Biology Society (EMBC)*. (IEEE, 2015), pp. 3029–3032
101. E. Topol, *Deep Medicine: How Artificial Intelligence Can Make Healthcare Human Again* (Hachette UK, 2019)
102. S. Dash, B.R. Acharya, M. Mittal, A. Abraham, A. Kelemen, *Deep Learning Techniques for Biomedical and Health Informatics* (Springer, 2020)
103. A. Panesar, *Machine Learning and AI for Healthcare* (Apress, 2019)
104. M. Chang, *Artificial Intelligence for Drug Development, Precision Medicine, and Healthcare* (Chapman and Hall/CRC, 2020)

Chapter 4
Diagnosing Diabetic Retinopathy by Using a Blood Vessel Extraction Technique and a Convolutional Neural Network

As a critical relation with image processing and deep learning, it is a remarkable research way to work on medical images. As an important disease, diabetic retinopathy has the potential of being analyzed over medical images. Among adverse events associated with diabetes, there is the diabetic retinopathy as resulting to visual impairment if treatment deficiencies are not solved in long-term. Diabetic retinopathy (DR) is a critical eye disease as a result of the diabetes and is the most widely-seen factor of blindness for the countries in the developed-state. One in three diabetic individuals has symptoms of DR, and unfortunately this is a very serious threat to their vision. Naturally, early diagnosis and also treatments are very vital to prevent patients against effects or at least to slow the progression of DR. Therefore, a mass screening of diabetic patients is extremely important [1–3].

It is remarkable that World Health Organization (WHO) has been announcing as well as reporting guidelines and diabetes-related developments for the diagnosis and classification of diabetes data for more than fifty years. WHO and the International Diabetes Federation (IDF) publish reviews and updates at different periods to identify, diagnose and classify diabetes and its complications. The IDF reported that in 2013 there were 385 million diabetes patients worldwide, most of which were type-2 diabetes. That value is estimated to reach around total of 592 million by 2035. According to WHO statistics, globally, 2% of diabetic patients with disease have been blinded for more than 15-year period, and 10% have high-level visual impairment, and also 32% have abnormal retinopathy [4–7].

The costs (in terms of economic, medical, and also social) of diabetes are a major public problem and diabetes is at the fourth row as the cause of deaths worldwide [6]. It is noteworthy also that devastating cardiovascular macro-micro problems associated with diabetes rises significant reductions in the context of quality-level of life as well as the expectancy [8]. Therefore, the definition, diagnosis and classification of diabetes is very important, and many scientists, especially under the guidance of WHO and IDF, are working on these issues. However, manual ratings may not always give accurate results because they require good experience and expertise. Therefore,

© The Editor(s) (if applicable) and The Author(s), under exclusive license to Springer Nature Singapore Pte Ltd. 2021
U. Kose et al., *Deep Learning for Medical Decision Support Systems*,
Studies in Computational Intelligence 909,
https://doi.org/10.1007/978-981-15-6325-6_4

many studies have been carried out to develop computer-assisted diagnostic systems to assist eye specialists. Much of the related efforts have been spent for development of reliable computerized scanning systems by classifying color fundus images in most of these studies [1–3].

Diabetic retinopathy (DR) is briefly as a result of abnormalities of blood vessels, which can be seen as a vascular complication. It therefore causes diabetics to have a risk of being blind 25 times more, according to the people having no diabetes. It is remarkable that 40.3% of the patients over the age of 40 have DR. There are four stages of DR [9]:

- **Mild proliferative retinopathy**: Here, the microaneurysms occur and may cause bleeding or hard exudates.
- **Moderately non-proliferative retinopathy**: At this stage, the cotton wool stains occur because retinal cultivation is deprived.
- **Severe proliferative retinopathy**: Here at the third stage, the blood supply can restrict many areas of the retina and the some of blood vessels.
- **Proliferative retinopathy**: At that final stage, vitreous gel accordingly flows to the eye and then the blood vessels cannot ensure adequate flow of the blood. Eventually, the vision may be lost and that state may go towards even blindness.

In general, the DR is classified with five types, as according the presence of clinical features. These are respectively (1) the mild-Non-Proliferative Diabetic Retinopathy (NPDR), (2) the moderate NPDR, (3) the severe NPDR, (4) PDR, and (5) the Macular Edema (ME) [10]. Figure 4.1 shows normal retina and three types of DR images such as normal retina, macular edema (ME), proliferative diabetic retinopathy (PDR), and non-proliferative diabetic retinopathy (NPDR) in Messidor retinal fundus database.

Exudates are indications for the diagnosis of diabetic ME and can be seen with a white or yellow-like color as a result of the fat and proteins from microaneurysm. Size varies according to the shapes and also location. These are usually take place in lines or clusters or surround the microaneurysms [9]. The diagnosis of DR is generally made use of these features.

In this chapter, the diagnosis of DR with a deep learning method by using the color retinal fundus images obtained from Messidor Database was investigated and the performance of convolutional neural network was emphasized. Then, the materials and methods used in the diagnostic process were explained. After giving the basic features of the application, the findings and the discussions about the results were given.

4.1 Related Works

Because of the importance of DR, many studies have been conducted for its diagnosis. In these studies, retinal color fundus images and a Convolution Neural Network as a deep learning method (CNN) are widely used. Since the inputs of automated DR diagnosis systems are the retinal fundus images, the system inputs are improved by

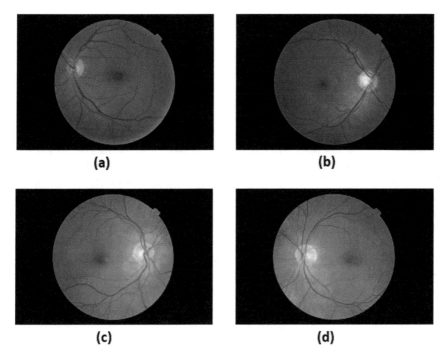

Fig. 4.1 a Healthy retina, **b** the macular edema (ME), **c** the proliferative DR (PDR), and **d** the non-proliferative DR (NPDR)

using image preprocessing and image processing techniques. The classification is then performed with CNN or enhanced models. Recent examples of DR detection with deep learning are given below.

Sahlsten and his colleagues in their study, have proposed a system for diagnosing DR using CNN. In addition, for five different screening and clinical grading systems in the classification of diabetic retinopathy and macular edema, they provided the results of studies to accurately classify images according to clinical five-grade diabetic retinopathy [11].

Arcadu et al. unlike many other studies, they conducted a study on the predictive level of DR. In this study, they proposed an approach to predict the progression of DR by CNN using color fundus images as input get from a patient with DR. Here, the solution-method is for predicting future DR progression regarding the 2-stage worsening of the Early Treatment Diabetic Retinopathy Severity Scale of Diabetic Retinopathy. They attempted to estimate the severity of DR, assessed at 6, 12, and 24 month's periods. They also developed correlation maps for the indicated periods. These maps highlight the areas in which the CNN model focuses attention on how to classify a particular query image. This study discusses the feasibility and efficiency of predicting future DR progression using fundus images of a patient from a single visit [12].

Chandrakumar and Kathirvel run a three-stage solution approach for the diagnosis of DR. The first stage is the increased data stage obtained by taking the fundus images from different data sets under different cameras with different field of view, sharpness, blurring, contrast and different image sizes. In the second stage, image preprocessing was performed. At this stage, the images were first converted to gray scale, then to the L model and then to binary image. In the last stage, the classification was performed with CNN which have 6 layers. They have obtained an overall accuracy around 94% for detecting the diabetic retinopathy stages in the context of the datasets of the STARE, and the DRIVE [13]. In another study using an augmented data stage was made Gao and his colleagues. In their study, dataset construction stage consisted of 8 different steps as: (1) collection, (2) annotation, (3) preprocessing, (4) augmentation, (5) model setting-up, (6) evaluation, (7) deployment of the model, and finally (8) clinical evaluation. Evaluation of the model, which was the Classification with CNN models of this dataset, was made with 7 databases. These database were respectively Digital Retinal Images for Vessel Extraction (DRIVE) dataset, Standard Diabetic Retinopathy Database Calibration Level 0/1 (DIARETDB0-DIARETDB1) dataset, Structured Analysis of the Retina (the STARE) dataset, Methods to Evaluate Segmentation and Indexing techniques in the field of Retinal Ophthalmology (the MESSIDOR) dataset, Retinal Vessel Image set for Estimation of Widths (the REVIEW) dataset, Kaggle Diabetic Retinopathy dataset, and the E-ophtha dataset. The CNN models were Resnet-18, Resnet-101, VGG-19, Inception@4, and InceptionV3. From the obtained results, it was seen that the adapted Inception@4 model and the Inception-V3 model both performed better than all other models [14].

In particular, convolutional neural networks (CNNs) have been developed to classify images and have been widely used in DR diagnostic studies. For example, Deperlioglu and Kose used a practical image processing method to improve retinal fundus images including HSV, V transformation algorithm and histogram equalization techniques. They classified the images with CNN [15]. Hemant and his colleagues used image processing that contains the histogram equalization technique (HE) as well as the contrast limited adaptive histogram equalization technique (CLAHE), and finally a CNN for the classification [16]. Pratt et al. recommended a CNN to diagnose DR from digital images of fundus and classify successfully enough the severity of DR. They employed CNN architecture and also a data enhancement process that can see complex features (such as Micro-aneurysms, exudate and bleeding in the retina), as took place within the classification phase. As a result, they have developed a diagnosis system which works automatic and don't need a user input [17].

Dutta et al. in their study, an automatic information model was proposed to identify the main precursors of DR from fundus images containing diabetic retinopathy. Backpropagation Artificial Neural Network, Deep Neural Network (DNN) and Convolution Neural Network (CNN) were used for classification. The weighted Fuzzy C-average algorithm was used to define the thresholds related to the target class. The model will help to identify the appropriate degree of severity of diabetic retinopathy images. With the proposed model, weights of the patient's eye giving the severity level were calculated. Deep Learning models have been more successful in classifying features such as blood vessels, fluid dripping, exudates, hemorrhages and micro aneurysms [18].

In another study, performances of convolutional neural network (CNN) models on fundus images (in colorful form) for recognition of diabetic retinopathy staging have been demonstrated. Prior to image preprocessing in the study, images were cropped using Otsu's method to isolate the circular image of the retina. The images were then normalized to contrast adjustment, CLAHE filtering algorithm. In the study using GoogLeNet and AlexNet models from ImageNet, the GoogLeNet model reached to the highest rates for both sensitivity, and the specificity [19].

As can be seen from the examples given above, there are several diagnostic methods for DR diagnosis from color retinal images of fundus have made with the different image processing techniques and the different CNN models.

4.2 Materials and Methods

As can be seen from the examples given in the previous section, many studies have been conducted with deep learning for the diagnosis of DR using retinal fundus images. In these studies, different image processing techniques and hybrid methods with CNN models are generally used. The aim of this study is to show that classification can be made easily by using image processing method to extract blood vessels within the retinal image and traditional convolutional neural network. Thus, an effective diagnosis could be made. The process steps or the flow chart of the developed method were given in Fig. 4.2.

As shown in the flow chart, 250 color fundus images from the public Messidor database were used in the application. For ensuring lower memory requirement in the classification process, the sizes of the images were changed and reduced from 1448×2240 to 149×224 pixels. The image was then converted from the RGB color space to Gray format. Then, by using Kirsch's Template method, retinal blood vessels were extracted and image processing was completed. The classification was then performed with 8-layers CNN. For all classification study, MATLAB r2017a software was used.

4.2.1 Messidor Dataset

MESSIDOR represents the Methods for Evaluating Segmentation and Indexing Techniques in the Retinal Ophthalmology (in French) section. The Messidor database was created during the Messidor project to facilitate studies on computer-aided diagnosis of diabetic retinopathy from color retinal fundus images and to evaluate different lesion segmentation methods. In this study, the reason for using this

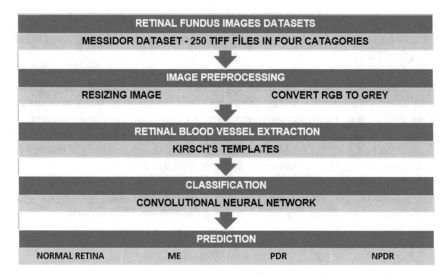

Fig. 4.2 Flow chart regarding the developed method

database, which has been open to the public for ten years, is to indicate the DR levels of retinal fundus images [20–22].

Images obtaining processes for the database is as follows: Three departments of ophthalmologic gathered totally 1200 eye-fundus images (in colorful forms) of the posterior pole by using a colored camera of 3CCD (on a Topcon TRC NW6 non-mydriatic retinograph with 45° area to view). Here, the corresponding images were got over a 8-bit per color plane at one of the 2240 * 1488, 1440 * 960, or 2304 * 1536 pixels. 800 images with pupil dilation, and also a total of 400 images with no dilation (done with one drop Tropicamide at 0.5%) were get eventually [16, 20–22]. These images were classified by the experts as considering four different levels. In the context of the levels, (1) the Risk 0 correspond to non-DR images, (2) the Risk 1 means the mild DR, (3) the Risk 2 to moderate DR, and finally, (4) the Risk 3 corresponds to an advanced stage of DR. In this study, the degree of retinopathy given in the database was used as a reference. The definition of the number of images for each level is given in Table 4.1 [23, 24].

Table 4.1 Retinopathy grade in Messidor database

Grade	Description	Number of images
R1	$(N_{MA} = 0)$ AND $(N_{HE} = 0)$	546
R2	$(0 < N_{MA} \leq 5)$ AND $(N_{HE} = 0)$	153
R3	$(5 < N_{MA} < 15)$ AND $(0 < N_{HE} < 5)$ AND $(N_{NV} = 0)$	247
R4	$(N_{MA} \geq 15)$ OR $(N_{HE} \geq 5)$ OR $(N_{NV} > 0)$	254

N_{MA}, N_{HE}, N_{NV}: number of MAs, HEs and neovessels (NV), respectively

4.2.2 Image Processing

Image processing method contains the resizing retinal image and the extracting the related vessels from each of the target image of the retina. Figure 4.3 represents the general steps done within that image processing phase.

In the image processing stage, retinal fundus images, which were primarily 1488 × 2240 pixels in size, were reduced to 149 × 224 pixels. The aim is to reduce the amount of memory that images require only during classification. After resizing, the RGB image in TIFF format was converted to GRAY image.

Retinal vessels are often referred to as veins and arteries. Here, the central retinal artery and also vein are close to each other (normally) in the center of the optic disc. Blood vessels are the most obvious in the green component. Knowledge of the structure of blood vessels can allows rating the severity level of the diseases and can also play an important role during the operation. At this point, two different strategies have been employed for detecting the blood vessels in human image. These are respectively edge detection, and the tracking as requiring prior information about the starting position in the image [25].

Fig. 4.3 The process steps of the image processing

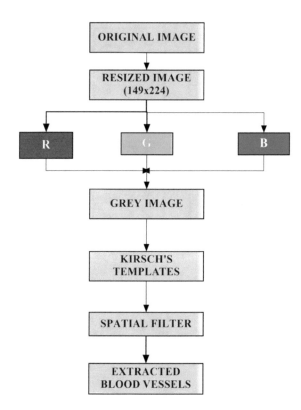

Edge detection was used in this study. Kirsch's Template method, one of the edge detection methods, was run for extraction of the blood vessels in the general retinal fundus image [26]. Kirsch's Template method has been used in many applications for ensuring extracting of the blood vessels. Since the Kirsch operator can adjust the threshold (automatically), by considering the character of the image, the Kirsch gradient operator is selected to subtract the contour of the object. That operator briefly ensures eight window templates (H1–H8). These eight window templates (H1–H8) are given in Fig. 4.4. Each template gives the largest response in a given direction relative to the edge directions. With the exception of the outermost column and the outermost row, each pixel and its eight 3×3 neighborhoods contain eight curves with these eight templates, respectively. So each pixel has eight outputs, eight templates are selected as the value at this location. The gray value of a P (i, j) point and the eight neighborhoods in the image are shown as in Fig. 4.4 [25, 27]. In practice, the scale factor was taken as 1/15.

The Kirsch's Template operator receives a single core mask and rotates 450 images of 8 compass directions, such as North, Northwest, South, Southwest, East, Northeast, Southeast, and West. The edge size is get as the maximum size in all of the

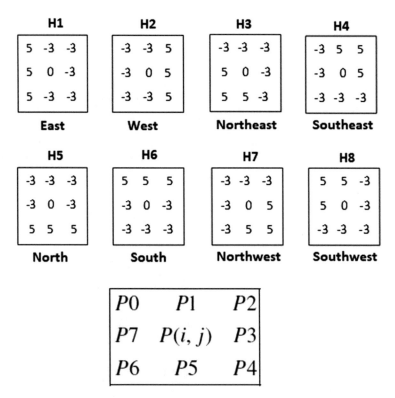

Fig. 4.4 The eight templates of the Kirsch operator and the gray value of a point and its eight neighborhoods P(*i, j*)

directions. Each pixel of the images uses these 8 masking to make the folds. Each masking responds greatly to a particular edge direction, the maximum value of 8 directions being determined as the output value of this point. The masking sequence number of the maximum value generates the code for the edge direction [28]. Finally, spatial filtering of the input retinal image is done in different directions with Kirsch Templates. Followed by thresholding, results in the extracted blood vessels. The threshold value that can be adjusted to fine tune the output is set to 10 in this application. In order not to increase the extra workload during the image processing phase, no operations such as filtering or morphological erosion were performed.

4.2.3 Classification with Convolutional Neural Network

In practice, Convolutional neural network (CNN) was used to diagnose levels of DR or healthy person by classifying the images in the dataset. The general structure of CNN is briefly explained below.

The Convolutional Neural Network (CNN) which is one of the deep learning technique is a kind of feedforward neural network of the connection model between neurons that responds to the overlapping regions of the individual neurons in image recognition. CNN uses a complex architecture of stacked layers that are particularly well adapted to classify images. CNN is robust and sensitive to every feature found in images, especially for classification studies with a high output classes. Figure 4.5 illustrates the basic structure of an example CNN [13].

Convolutional neural networks generally consist of one or more convolutional layers, which are a sub-sampling step. It then consists of one or more fully connected layers, such as a standard multilayer neural network. A CNN architecture is designed to take advantage of the 2D structure of two-dimensional (2D) image inputs. This is summed up by local connections and associated weights, leading to continuously changing properties. Another benefit of CNNs is that they have less training and easier parameters than networks that are completely connected to the same number

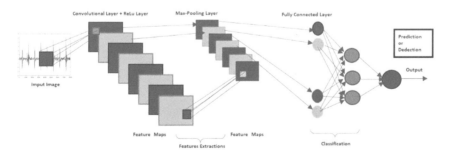

Fig. 4.5 The basic structure of an example CNN

of hidden nodes. CNNs use spatial-local correlation by applying a local binding pattern between neurons of adjacent layer [29].

4.2.4   Evaluation of Performance

Classification studies done in the context of medical employs different equations to evaluate the performance from different points. Accuracy, Precision, Recall, F-measure, specificity, and sensitivity are some of them and these equations-calculations are run for evaluating the precision of a used classification model [30].

Performance evaluators ensures important role in the classification tasks. The accuracy is most popular criteria and the proportion of correct decisions taken by a classifier. Sensitivity which is also called recall, figures out how much the related classifier is able to recognize the positive examples. Additionally, the specificity figures out how much the same classifier is able to recognize the negative examples. Precision is a really positive prediction rate of positive samples. It is known that there is a decreasing hyperbolic relationship between sensitivity and precision, and one way to deal with it is using ROC charts. A ROC graph is two-dimensional, in which the false positive ratio (1—specificity) is plotted on the horizontal axis and the precision is plotted on the vertical axis. Also, F-measure is the harmonic mean of sensitivity and precision [31]:

$$Accuracy = \frac{TP + TN}{TP + TN + FP + FN} \tag{4.1}$$

$$Sensitivity = \frac{TP}{TP + FN} \tag{4.2}$$

$$Specificity = \frac{TN}{FPTN + TN} \tag{4.3}$$

$$Precision = \frac{TP}{TP + FP} \tag{4.4}$$

$$Recall = Sensitivity \tag{4.5}$$

$$F\text{-}measure = 2 * \left[\frac{(Precision * Recall)}{(Precision + Recall)} \right] \tag{4.6}$$

In these Eqs. (4.1–4.6), TP, and the FP means respectively the total number regarding true positive, and the total number regarding false positive diagnosis. TN and FN the numbers of true negatives, and false negatives, respectively. FPTN also represents the number of false positives and it is calculated from negative samples in the results of classification.

For the classifier, accuracy refers to the accuracy of the correct diagnosis. The sensitivity ratio indicates how accurately the classifier defines the occurrence of the target class. The specificity ratio is used to define the classifier's ability to allocate the target class. Precision is a measure of the quality of precise or accurate results. Recall, also known as true positive rate and provides the proportion of positively defined positives in a test. The F-measure is also known as the F1 score and provides a metric of the accuracy of a test. It is the weighted harmonic mean of sensitivity and recall [32, 33].

4.3 Diagnosis Application

MATLAB r2017a software was used in all image processing and classification studies. In this application, randomly selected 200 color retinal fundus digital images from Messidor database were used to evaluate the introduced method within this study. The database comes with four different output classes as the normal retina, the macular edema (ME), the proliferative diabetic retinopathy (PDR), and the non-proliferative diabetic retinopathy (NPDR). 200 color retinal fundus digital images randomly selected from the Messidor database are divided as follows: 99 normal, 19 macular edema (ME), 27 proliferative diabetic retinopathy (PDR), and finally, 55 non-proliferative diabetic retinopathy (NPDR).

This 200 color retinal fundus digital image was processed as described image processing techniques in the previous section. Retinal vessel extraction was performed using Kirsch's Template method. The samples of extracted retinal vessel images obtained at the end of image processing is given in Fig. 4.6. In Fig. 4.6, the extracted blood vessels (a) is for 20051213_61892_0100_PP.tif image, and (b) is for 20051213_61951_0100_PP.tif image from Messidor Database. The classification stage was performed with these obtained images.

The extracted blood vessel images were classified by CNN. CNNs are a type of deep network that receives and processes image data with its label as an object. In this model, CNN has 8 layers. These layers are respectively image input layer, convolutional layer, ReLU layer, cross channel normalization layer, max pooling layer, fully connected layer, softmax layer and the classification (grading layer). Details of the related layers are given in Table 4.2.

Input Layer is used to specify the values of the image. In this study, the image values are $149 \times 224 \times 3$ and these numbers correspond to the height, width and RGB format of the images, respectively. Data transformations in this layer, such as data normalization or data enhancement, are based on the idea of random translation and the truncation of related data. Data conversion is often used to prevent overfitting and is done automatically at the beginning of the training process.

In this CNN model has one convolutional layer. The parameters of the convolutional layer are associated with the size of the network filtering. At this point, the filter

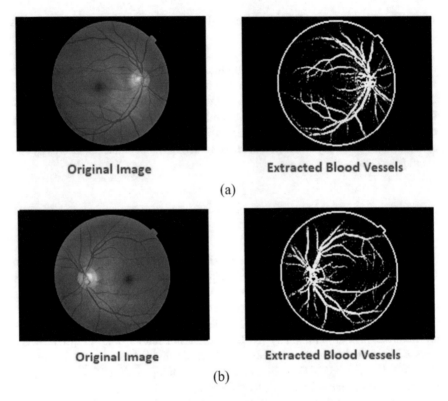

Fig. 4.6 The extracted blood vessels **a** for 20051213_61892_0100_PP.tif, **b** for 20051213_61951_0100_PP.tif image from Messidor database

Table 4.2 CNN layers and their properties

Order no	Layers	Properties
1	Input layer	[149 224 3]
2	Convolutional layer	(4, 16)
3	ReLU layer	–
4	Cross channel normalization layer	(2)
5	Maximum pool layer	(4, 'Stride', 3)
6	Fully connected layer	(numClasses, 'WLRF', 20, 'BLRF', 20)
7	Softmax layer	%89.47
8	Classification layer	%78.00

size was determined as 4, and the second parameter regarding the number of neurons determining the total feature maps and bound to the same region of the output as the number of filters, was selected 16.

Rectified Linear Unit (ReLU) layer is an activation function. A nonlinear activation function was provided by following the convolutional layer in the ReLU layer. Here, the function of rectified linear unit was run accordingly.

On the other hand, as one cross channel normalization layer was included in the CNN, the size of the channel window was 2, which corresponds to also channel window size for the normalization.

The maximum pooling layer is used for down sampling in order to reduce total number of the parameters and so that preventing from the issue of overfitting. Briefly, that layer returns the maximum values of the regions (rectangles) of the entries specified by the first argument pool size. In this model, the size of the rectangle is set to [3, 4]. The step function is also used to determine the step size while the image is thoroughly scanned by the exercise function.

The fully connected layer collects all relevant properties that previously placed layers have learned about the image to identify larger patterns. To classify on these, the last of the fully connected layer collects them. Therefore, the output size parameter on the last layer that is fully connected is set to the number of classes in the target table. The database contains four output classes such as normal retina, macular edema (ME), proliferative diabetic retinopathy (PDR), and non-proliferative diabetic retinopathy (NPDR). For this reason, the number of output classes (numClasses) is 4.

The last layer in the CNN model is the classification layer. In the context of classification applications, that fully connected layer is often based on the softmax activation function. This layer estimates using the possibilities returned by the softmax activation function for each entry to mutually assign one of the custom classes.

For the proposed CNN model, a sample screen shot was given Fig. 4.7. This Fig. 4.7 also shows obtained values at the end of classification trial.

In the classification application, randomly selected 160 images (80% of samples) from Messidor Retinal Fundus Image Dataset were used as training data and 40 images (20% of samples) were used test data. The classification study was repeated 20 times for randomly selected different training and test data.

In the proposed CNN model, the maximum epoch value was set 200 epochs and the number of hidden layers was 10. In the classification application, randomly selected 80% samples (160 images) from Messidor Retinal Fundus Image Dataset were used as training data and 20% samples (40 images) were used test data. The classification study was repeated 20 times for randomly selected different training and test data.

4.4 Results and Discussion

The experimental results were assessed with performance evaluation criterias such as accuracy, specificity, sensitivity, precision, recall, and the F-measure.

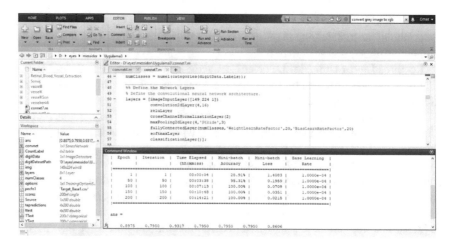

Fig. 4.7 A sample screen shot for the proposed CNN model

The obtained performance values via 20 classification trials were given in Table 4.3, which were the accuracy, specificity, sensitivity, precision, recall, and F-measure.

As can be seen from Table 4.3, quite high values were obtained. In order to better interpret the performance criteria of the classification trials, the lowest, the average and the highest values for each criterion are given in Table 4.4.

As can be seen from Table 4.4, the lowest classification accuracy rate was 87.25%, the average classification accuracy rate was 89.84%, and the highest classification accuracy rate was 91.50%. The lowest classification sensitivity and recall rates were 74.5%, the average classification sensitivity and recall rates were 79.68%, and the highest classification sensitivity and recall rates were 83.0%. The lowest classification specificity rate was 91.5%, the average classification specificity rate was 93.23%, and the highest classification specificity rate was 94.33%.

The lowest classification precision and F-measure rates were 74.5%, the average classification precision and F-measure rates were 79.68%, and the highest classification precision and F-measure rates were 83.3%.

Classification studies for the Messidor dataset with CNN have high accuracy, sensitivity and specificity rates. The performance criterias of the proposed model were compared with previous studies used the same database to evaluate its performance. Table 4.5 reports the obtained findings in this manner.

The highest accuracy, sensitivity and specificity values were obtained by image processing and CNN approaches. Obtaining very different results in applications with the same CNN model for the same database [this study, 15, 16] shows the importance of image processing. The values obtained in blood vessel extraction and CNN application proposed in this study are still above the traditional methods and average values.

Table 4.3 The obtained performance criterias in the 20 classification trials

Trial no	Accuracy	Sensitivity	Specificity	Precision	Recall	F-measure
1	0.8725	0.7450	0.9150	0.7450	0.7450	0.7450
2	0.8950	0.7900	0.9300	0.7900	0.7900	0.7900
3	0.8950	0.7900	0.9300	0.7900	0.7900	0.7900
4	0.8900	0.7800	0.9267	0.7800	0.7800	0.7800
5	0.9050	0.8100	0.9367	0.8100	0.8100	0.8100
6	0.9100	0.8200	0.9400	0.8200	0.8200	0.8200
7	0.8950	0.7900	0.9300	0.7900	0.7900	0.7900
8	0.8925	0.7850	0.9283	0.7850	0.7850	0.7850
9	0.8975	0.7950	0.9317	0.7950	0.7950	0.7950
10	0.8950	0.7900	0.9300	0.7900	0.7900	0.7900
11	0.9150	0.8300	0.9433	0.8300	0.8300	0.8300
12	0.8775	0.7550	0.9183	0.7550	0.7550	0.7550
13	0.9050	0.8100	0.9367	0.8100	0.8100	0.8100
14	0.9050	0.8100	0.9367	0.8100	0.8100	0.8100
15	0.9150	0.8300	0.9433	0.8300	0.8300	0.8300
16	0.8950	0.7900	0.9300	0.7900	0.7900	0.7900
17	0.9050	0.8100	0.9367	0.8100	0.8100	0.8100
18	0.9100	0.8200	0.9400	0.8200	0.8200	0.8200
19	0.9150	0.8300	0.9433	0.8300	0.8300	0.8300
20	0.8775	0.7550	0.9183	0.7550	0.7550	0.7550
Average	0.8984	0.7968	0.9323	0.7968	0.7968	0.7968

Table 4.4 The lowest, the average and the highest values of performance criterias

Criteria	Lowest	Average	Highest
Accuracy	0.8725	0.8984	0.9150
Sensitivity	0.7450	0.7968	0.8300
Specificity	0.9150	0.9323	0.9433
Precision	0.7450	0.7968	0.8300
Recall	0.7450	0.7968	0.8300
F-measure	0.7450	0.7968	0.8300

The obtained high sensitivity shows that the developed model accurately defines the formation of the target class. The obtained high specificity ratio shows that the developed model has a very high ability to allocate the target class. F-measure is the harmonic mean of the classifier and its recall. In most cases, there is a balance between precision and recall. If you optimize the classifier to increase one and remove the other, the harmonic average decreases rapidly. However, when both sensitivity

Table 4.5 The comparison of classification accuracies, sensitivities, and specificities

Method	Accuracy	Sensitivity	Specificity
Vessel extraction and CNN (this study)	0.8984	0.7968	0.9323
Image processing and CNN [15]	0.9730	–	–
Image processing and CNN [16]	0.9700	**0.9400**	**0.9800**
Image processing and CNN [34]	0.9600	1	0.9000
Deep neural network (DNN) [35]	**0.9800****	0.9000	0.9600
Ensemble-based framework [2]	0.8200	0.7600	0.8800
Bag of words model [3]	0.9440	0.9400	–
Particle swarm optimization and the fuzzy C-means [36]	0.9450	0.9100	0.9800
Fractal analysis and K-nearest neighbor (KNN) [37]	0.8917	–	–
Texture features, and support vector machine (SVM) [38]	0.8520	0.8950	0.972
Marker-controlled watershed transformation [39]	0.8520	0.8090	0.9020

Best values are in bold
**ROC value

and recall are equal, it is the largest. If the F-measure is very high, the classifier is in very good condition.

This study demonstrated that CNN can detect reproducible diabetic retinopathy with a sensitivity and specificity of close to 80 and 90% or higher for the Messidor database. It can successfully detect four different types of images in the database.

4.5 Summary

Diabetic retinopathy is known as a critical-vital medical problem associated with the diabetes. That's because it causes visual impairment if the treatment is not performed properly in long-term. Diabetic retinopathy (DR) is a serious eye disease caused by diabetes and is the most common cause of blindness in developed countries. One in three diabetic individuals has symptoms of DR, and unfortunately this is a very serious threat to their vision. Naturally, early diagnosis and treatment are very important to prevent patients from being affected or at least slow the progression of DR. Therefore, mass screening of diabetic patients is extremely important.

Diabetic retinopathy (DR) is a result of the abnormalities of blood vessels, which is known as a vascular complication. It therefore causes diabetics resulting to a risk of blindness 25 times higher than people with no disease of the diabetes. 40.3% of patients over the age of 40 have DR. There are four stages of DR [9]:

- **Mild proliferative retinopathy**: At the first stage, the microaneurysms occur and may cause bleeding or hard exudates.
- **Moderately non-proliferative retinopathy**: At this second stage, the cotton wool stains occur because retinal cultivation is deprived.

- **Severe proliferative retinopathy**: Here at the third stage, the blood supply can restrict many areas of the retina and several blood vessels.
- **Proliferative retinopathy**: At that final stage, vitreous gel accordingly flows to the eye and then the blood vessels cannot ensure adequate flow of the blood. Eventually, the vision may be lost and that state may go towards even blindness.

Generally, the DR is observed with five different types, by analyzing the presence of clinical features. These are respectively mild Non-Proliferative Diabetic Retinopathy (NPDR), moderate NPDR, severe NPDR, PDR and Macular Edema (ME) [10]. Figure 4.1 shows normal retina and three types of DR images such as normal retina, macular edema (ME), proliferative diabetic retinopathy (PDR), and non-proliferative diabetic retinopathy (NPDR) in Messidor retinal fundus database.

Because of the importance of DR, many studies have been conducted for its diagnosis. In these studies, retinal color fundus images and a Convolution Neural Network as a deep learning method (CNN) were widely used. Since the inputs of automated DR diagnosis systems are the retinal fundus images, the system inputs are improved by using image preprocessing and image processing techniques. The classification is then performed with CNN or enhanced models.

That 200 retinal fundus (colorful) digital image was processed as described image processing techniques in the previous section. Retinal vessel extraction was performed using Kirsch's Template method. The extracted blood vessel images were classified by CNN. CNNs are a type of deep network that receives and processes image data with its label as an object. In this model, CNN has 8 layers. These layers are respectively image input layer, convolutional layer, ReLU layer, cross channel normalization layer, max pooling layer, fully connected layer, softmax layer and grading (classification layer).

The experimental results were assessed with performance evaluation criterias such as accuracy, specificity, sensitivity, precision, recall, and F-measure, obtained from trials. When performance criterias are compared with previous studies used Messidor dataset, the highest accuracy, sensitivity and specificity values have obtained by image processing and CNN approaches. Obtaining very different results in applications with the same CNN model for the same database [this study, 15, 16] shows the importance of image processing. The values obtained in blood vessel extraction and CNN application proposed in this study are still above the traditional methods and average.

This study demonstrated that CNN can detect reproducible diabetic retinopathy with a sensitivity and specificity of close to 80 and 90% or higher for the Messidor database. It can successfully detect four different types of images in the database.

In addition to medical image applications, deep learning is effective on processing sound data, too. Since a medical decision support system should be able to deal with multimedia-type data, it is important to diagnose diseases by using sound data. As associated with a serious disease: Parkinson's, the next Chap. 5 is devoted to a explain of such a research.

4.6   Further Learning

In order to investigate in detail, the characteristics of CNN techniques and methods, [29] could be seen.

The articles in [2, 3, 36–39] could be examined to see the applications and performances of diagnosis DR with different traditional AI techniques.

References [2, 9, 24, 40, 41] can be examined for a model of DR detection using different methods, including procedures such as extraction candidate lesions, feature set formulation, and classification.

To see the details of Kirsch's template method, which is the edge selection method, [14, 25, 28] can be examined. It can also be examined for applications in color fundus images [42, 43].

References

1. Ö. Deperlıoğlu, U. Köse, Diagnosis of diabetic retinopathy by using image processing and convolutional neural network, in *2018 2nd International Symposium on Multidisciplinary Studies and Innovative Technologies (ISMSIT)*, Oct 2018 (IEEE), pp. 1–5
2. B. Antal, A. Hajdu, An ensemble-based system for microaneurysm detection and diabetic retinopathy grading. IEEE Trans. Biomed. Eng. **59**(6), 1720–1726 (2012)
3. M. Islam, A.V. Dinh, K.A. Wahid, Automated diabetic retinopathy detection using bag of words approach. J. Biomed. Sci. Eng. **10**, 86–96 (2017)
4. World Health Organization and International Diabetes Federation, *Definition and diagnosis of diabetes mellitus and intermediate hyperglycemia* [Report of World Health Organization and International Diabetes Federation] (2005)
5. International Diabetes Federation, *Diabetes Atlas*, 6th edn. (Brussels, Belgium, 2013), https://www.idf.org/sites/default/files/EN_6E_Atlas_Full_0.pdf. Son erişim 23 Ocak 2018
6. International Diabetes Federation, *Diabetes Atlas*, 4th edn. (Brussels, Belgium, 2009), Available from https://www.idf.org/sites/default/files/IDF-Diabetes-Atlas-4th-edition.pdf. Cited 23 June 2018
7. S. Wild, G. Roglic, A. Green, R. Sicree, H. King, Global prevalence of diabetes: estimates for the year 2000 and projections for 2030. Diabetes Care **27**(5), 1047–1053 (2004)
8. A.I. Veresiu, C.I. Bondor, B. Florea, E.J. Vinik, A.I. Vinik, N.A. Gâvan, Detection of undisclosed neuropathy and assessment of its impact on quality of life: a survey in 25,000 Romanian patients with diabetes. J. Diabetes Complicat. **29**, 644–649 (2015)
9. W. Luangruangrong, P. Kulkasem, S. Rasmequan, A. Rodtook, K. Chinnasarn, Automatic exudates detection in retinal images using efficient integrated approaches, in *Signal and Information Processing Association Annual Summit and Conference (APSIPA), 2014 Asia-Pacific*, Dec 2014 (IEEE), pp. 1–5
10. M.R.K. Mookiah et al., Computer-aided diagnosis of diabetic retinopathy: a review. Comput. Biol. Med. **43**(12), 2136–2155 (2013)
11. J. Sahlsten, J. Jaskari, J. Kivinen, L. Turunen, E. Jaanio, K. Hietala, K. Kaski, Deep learning fundus image analysis for diabetic retinopathy and macular edema grading (2019). arXiv preprint arXiv:1904.08764
12. F. Arcadu, F. Benmansour, A. Maunz, J. Willis, Z. Haskova, M. Prunotto, Deep learning algorithm predicts diabetic retinopathy progression in individual patients. NPJ Digit. Med. **2**(1), 1–9 (2019)
13. T. Chandrakumar, R. Kathirvel, Classifying diabetic retinopathy using deep learning architecture. Int. J. Eng. Res. Technol. **5**(6), 19–24 (2016)

14. Z. Gao, J. Li, J. Guo, Y. Chen, Z. Yi, J. Zhong, Diagnosis of diabetic retinopathy using deep neural networks. IEEE Access **7**, 3360–3370 (2018)
15. O. Deperlıoglu, U. Kose, Diagnosis of diabetic retinopathy by using image processing and convolutional neural network, in *2nd International Symposium on Multidisciplinary Studies and Innovative Technologies (ISMSIT)* (IEEE, 2018)
16. D.J. Hemanth, O. Deperlioglu, U. Kose, An enhanced diabetic retinopathy detection and classification approach using deep convolutional neural network. Neural Comput. Appl. (2019). https://doi.org/10.1007/s00521-018-03974-0
17. H. Pratt et al., Convolutional neural networks for diabetic retinopathy. Procedia Comput. Sci. **90**, 200–205 (2016)
18. S. Dutta, B.C. Manideep, S.M. Basha, R.D. Caytiles, N.C.S.N. Iyengar, Classification of diabetic retinopathy images by using deep learning models. Int. J. Grid Distrib. Comput. **11**(1), 89–106 (2018)
19. C. Lam, D. Yi, M. Guo, T. Lindsey, Automated detection of diabetic retinopathy using deep learning. AMIA Summits Transl. Sci. Proc. **2018**, 147 (2018)
20. MESSIDOR, *Methods to evaluate segmentation and indexing techniques in the field of retinal ophthalmology*. TECHNO-VISION Project. [Online]. Available: http://messidor.crihan.fr/
21. E. Decencière, Feedback on a publicly distributed image database: the Messidor database. Image Anal. Stereol. **33**, 231–234 (2014). https://doi.org/10.5566/ias.1155
22. The Messidor Database, http://www.adcis.net/en/third-party/messidor/. Last access 15 Jan 2020
23. L. Seoud, J. Chelbi, F. Cheriet, Automatic grading of diabetic retinopathy on a public database, in *Proceedings of the Ophthalmic Medical Image Analysis Second International Workshop, OMIA 2015*, ed. by X. Chen, M.K. Garvin, J.J. Liu, E. Trusso, Y. Xu, MICCAI 2015, Munich, Germany, 9 Oct 2015, pp. 97–104. Available from https://doi.org/10.17077/omia.1032
24. C. Agurto, V. Murray, E. Barriga, S. Murillo, M. Pattichis, H. Davis, P. Soliz, Multiscale AM-FM methods for diabetic retinopathy lesion detection. IEEE Trans. Med. Imaging **29**(2), 502–512 (2010)
25. H. Li, O. Chutatape, Fundus image features extraction, in *Proceedings of the 22nd Annual International Conference of the IEEE Engineering in Medicine and Biology Society (Cat. No. 00CH37143)*, vol. 4, July 2000 (IEEE), pp. 3071–3073
26. R.A. Kirsch, Computer determination of the constituent structure of biological images. Comput. Biomed. Res. **4**(3), 315–328 (1971)
27. P. Gao, X. Sun, W. Wang, Moving object detection based on Kirsch operator combined with optical flow, in *2010 International Conference on Image Analysis and Signal Processing*, Apr 2010 (IEEE), pp. 620–624
28. A. Venmathi, E. Ganesh, N. Kumaratharan, Kirsch compass Kernel edge detection algorithm for micro calcification clusters in mammograms. Middle-East J. Sci. Res. **24**(4), 1530–1535 (2016)
29. Convolutional Neural Networks (LeNet), http://deeplearning.net/tutorial/lenet.html. Last accessed 10.01.2018
30. W. Zhang, J. Han, S. Deng, Heart sound classification based on scaled spectrogram and tensor decomposition. Biomed. Signal Process. Control **32**, 20–28 (2017)
31. R.P. Espíndola, N.F.F. Ebecken, On extending f-measure and g-mean metrics to multi-class problems. WIT Trans. Inf. Commun. Technol. **35** (2005)
32. O. Deperlioglu, Classification of phonocardiograms with convolutional neural networks. BRAIN Broad Res. Artif. Intell. Neurosci. **9**(2), 23–33 (2018)
33. Q.-A. Mubarak, M.U. Akram, A. Shaukat, F. Hussain, S.G. Khawaja, W.H. Butt, Analysis of PCG signals using quality assessment and homomorphic filters for localization and classification of heart sounds. Comput. Methods Programs Biomed. (2018). https://doi.org/10.1016/j.cmpb.2018.07.006
34. L.R. Sudha, S. Thirupurasundari, Analysis and detection of haemorrhages and exudates in retinal images. Int. J. Sci. Res. Publ. **4**(3), 1–5 (2014)

35. N. Ramachandran, S.C. Hong, M.J. Sime, G.A. Wilson, Diabetic retinopathy screening using deep neural network. Clin. Exp. Ophthalmol. **46**, 412–416 (2018)
36. K.S. Sreejini, V.K. Govindan, Severity grading of DME from retina images: a combination of PSO and FCM with Bayes classifier. Int. J. Comput. Appl. **81**(16), 11–17 (2013)
37. D.W. Safitri, D. Juniati, Classification of diabetic retinopathy using fractal dimension analysis of eye fundus image. AIP Conf. Proc. **1867**, 020011-1–020011-11 (2017). https://doi.org/10.1063/1.4994414
38. U.R. Acharya, E.Y.K. Ng, J.H. Tan et al., An integrated index for the identification of diabetic retinopathy stages using texture parameters. J. Med. Syst. **36**(3), 2011–2020 (2012). https://doi.org/10.1007/s10916-011-9663-8
39. S.T. Lim, W.M.D.W. Zaki, A. Hussain, S.L. Lim, S. Kusavalan, Automatic classification of diabetic macular edama in fundus image. IEEE Colloq. Human. Sci. Eng. **5–6**, 1–4 (2011)
40. M.U. Akram, S. Khalid, A. Tariq, S.A. Khan, F. Azam, Detection and classification of retinal lesions for grading of diabetic retinopathy. Comput. Biol. Med. **45**, 161–171 (2014)
41. M.R.K. Mookiah, U.R. Acharya, C.K. Chua, C.M. Lim, E.Y.K. Ng, A. Laude, Computer-aided diagnosis of diabetic retinopathy: a review. Comput. Biol. Med. **43**(12), 2136–2155 (2013)
42. S. Badsha, A.W. Reza, K.G. Tan, K. Dimyati, A new blood vessel extraction technique using edge enhancement and object classification. J. Digit. Imaging **26**(6), 1107–1115 (2013)
43. A. Banumathi, R.K. Devi, V.A. Kumar, Performance analysis of matched filter techniques for automated detection of blood vessels in retinal images, in *TENCON 2003. Conference on Convergent Technologies for Asia-Pacific Region*, vol. 2, Oct 2003 (IEEE), pp. 543–546

Chapter 5
Diagnosing Parkinson by Using Deep Autoencoder Neural Network

The deep learning is strong on not only images (as explained in the previous Chap. 4) but also on sound-type data. It is possible to show that in a serious disease called as Parkinson's disease (PD). PD is a degenerative disease of the central nervous system. As coming after the Alzheimer's disease, PD is known among critical common neurodegenerative diseases. The number of people with PD worldwide is quite high and is rapidly increasing, especially in countries (developing) in the context of Asia. The Olmsted County (Mayo Clinic) has reported the life-time risk of Parkinson's disease at 2% for men. That value is 1.3 for women. It has been confirmed in many sources that the incidence of males is higher. It is stated that the number of PD patients will be doubled by 2030. Early diagnosis of PD disease can also reduce symptoms. Significant symptoms of PD are tremor, stiffness, slow motion, motor symptom asymmetry and impaired posture. In addition, phonation and speech disorders are common in the PD patients. As a result, PD is a chronic and progressive disorder of movements, and symptoms become worse over time. It is reported that almost 1 million people living in the US are an age with Parkinson's disease. The exact causes of the PD are unknown, so there is not any exact cure for now. However, treatment actions like medication and surgical intervention are available to manage the symptoms of male or female patients [1–6].

Parkinson's cause the breakdown and deaths appeared in the context of vital nerve cells called neurons in the brain, especially neurons called substantia nigra. These dying neurons may produce dopamine and that chemical can affect the part of the brain controlling movement as well as the coordination. Naturally, as PD progresses, the total dopamine amount in the brain will decrease so that causing a person to be unable to control movement normally. Here, tremor, stiffness, bradykinesia, and postural instability are known four main symptoms of the PD. Shivering means involuntary vibration for arms, hands, legs or jaws. Stiffness defines the flexibility to the limbs and the body whereas the slow motion corresponds to the bradykinesia. On the other hand, there may be the symptoms such as depression, and also emotional

© The Editor(s) (if applicable) and The Author(s), under exclusive license to Springer Nature Singapore Pte Ltd. 2021
U. Kose et al., *Deep Learning for Medical Decision Support Systems*,
Studies in Computational Intelligence 909,
https://doi.org/10.1007/978-981-15-6325-6_5

changes. There are also symptoms of swallowing, chewing and speech difficulties, urinary problems or constipation, skin problems and sleep disturbances [4–6].

Motoric dysfunction in every Parkinson's patient varies slightly in progress and response to medication. In general, accurate diagnosis requires a long process. It requires physicians to have significant experience in the disease, especially since various changes occur during a treatment. Recent research has shown that speech difficulties in 90% (as approximately) of the PD cases can be applied to differentiate between healthy and PD patients, even in the early stages of the disease [7]. Speech disorders in PD patients can be classified as dysphonia and dysarthria. Dysphonia is a deterioration in speech produce that may improve as a result of the disease progression. Dysarthria reflects that it cannot be jointed properly. Vocal pathology is caused by dysfunction of the laryngeal, articulator and respiratory muscles. Some studies have classified the general effects of speech disorder as wind, tremendous, treble, monotonous and muffled. Sound analysis techniques, such as spectrograms and electroglottographic (EGG) recordings of images of voice samples, can be used to identify disruptions in PD patients. For this, features obtained from patients's speech recordings under certain conditions and certain procedures are used [7–9].

In this chapter, the diagnosis of PD with a deep learning method by using the data obtained from Oxford Parkinson Diagnostic Data was investigated and the performance of deep learning was emphasized. Then, the materials and methods used in the diagnostic process were explained. After giving the basic features of the application, the findings and the discussions about the results were given.

5.1   Related Works

Until today, there are many studies with deep learning for the diagnosis of Parkinson's disease. In these studies, Electroencephalogram (EEG) signals, SPECT images or images obtained from diseased and healthy people were classified with Convolutional Neural Network. Rarely, deep neural network studies were also taking advantage of the sound features. Examples of studies for PD detection with deep learning were given below.

Martin colleagues in their study, using the CNN by evaluating the drawing movements have made the diagnosis of PD. In this study, feature extraction was performed with convolutional layers in CNN, and then totally bound layers were classified. Using the Digitized Graphics Tablet dataset, they obtained the PD Spiral Drawings dataset. At the end of the study they obtained a very efficient model with an accuracy of 96.5% [10]. Pereira and his colleagues have proposed a PD automatic diagnostic system which aims to learn the signal characteristics obtained from a signal obtained during the examination of the individual and a smart pen comprising a set of sensors capable of receiving information from handwritten dynamics. A CNN was used for classification. In their study, they achieved a 98% classification accuracy rate with CNN. They also stated that their dataset was first and could be used as an example [11].

Since PD is associated with brain abnormality, EEG signals are generally considered appropriate for early diagnosis. In their study, Oh et al. proposed an electroencephalogram (EEG) and CNN system to automatically detect PD. In the study, twenty normal subjects, and EEG signals belonging to twenty PD were used for evaluating the introduced system. The study uses a thirteen-layer CNN architecture to fully draw attention to the point features. The proposed model achieved 88.25% accuracy [12].

Dopaminergic degeneration is a pathological feature of PD, which can be evaluated by dopamine transporter imaging such as FP-CIT SPECT. Choi et al., considering this feature, have proposed a deep learning-based FP-CIT SPECT interpretation system for the diagnosis of PD. Trained with SPECT images of PD patients and normal individuals, this system uses CNN for a classification. Estimates obtained at the end of the study obtained high classification accuracy compared to the diagnostic results of the experts. They have also demonstrated that they can accurately interpret a typical PD subgroup dopaminergic deficit (SWEDD) FP-CIT SPECT [13]. Eskofier et al. using inertial units of measurement, they collected data from ten patients with idiopathic Parkinson's disease and classified them with CNN, and traditional methods such as boosting, decision trees, nearest neighbors and support vector machines. To test the proposed method, several engine-labeled tasks have been used by experts for a classification. The results they obtained with a CNN have encountered the results of traditional methods. Accordingly, it has been found that a CNN performs at least 4.6% better in terms of classification accuracy [14].

Magnetic Resonance Imaging (MRI) may also display structural changes in the brain, as caused by the dopamine deficiency in patients with the Parkinson's. In Sivaranjini and Sujatha study, they have made a classification process using a CNN structure AlexNet and healthy MR, and MR images with Parkinson's disease. With the proposed system, MR images were diagnosed with an accuracy rate of 88.9% [15]. Neuromelanin-sensitive magnetic-resonance-imaging (NMS-MRI) is here crucial for identifying abnormalities of substantia nigra pars compacta (SNc) as PD in Parkinson's disease (PD) because it is understood with loss of dopaminergic neurons in SNc. Today's techniques run an estimate of the contrast ratios of the SNc displayed on the NMS-MRI to differentiate PD patients from healthy controls. Shinde et al. used CNN to generate a prognostic and a diagnostic biomarker of PD from NMS-MRI. At the end of the study, they obtained 80% test accuracy and 85.7% test accuracy as a differential PD from atypical Parkinson's syndrome [16].

Ortiz et al. have developed a computer-assisted PD diagnostic system using 3D brain images. They used neural networks developed from CNN architecture such as LeNet and AlexNet for the classification process. They stated that the 3D brain images complicated the CNN structure because of the large amount of information. They suggested using isosurfaces to prevent this complex CNN structure from reducing the success of classification and to retain the most relevant information and to reduce others or excessive compliance. By using the proposed method, they made a classification of DaTScan images using LeNet and AlexNet CNN architectures. At the end of the study, the average classification accuracy rate was 95.1% and 97%, respectively. From the results, it is stated that the calculation of isosurfaces significantly reduces the complexity of the inputs and provides high classification accuracy. It can also be said that AlexNet has better results than LeNet for images with a lot of information [17].

Grover et al. Using the UCI's Parkinson's Telemonitoring Voice Data Set, they used a Deep Neural Network for PD prediction. They used python's 'TensorFlow' deep learning library to implement DNN. It is stated that the accuracy values obtained by the proposed method are better compared to the accuracy obtained in previous studies [18].

In the context of diagnosing Parkinson's disease via speech processing, there have been many research efforts in recent years. Muthumanickam et al. in their studies, have compared various machine learning, data mining, and deep learning algorithms such as K-nearest neighbor (kNN), Feedforward Back-Propagation Trained Artificial Neural Network (FBPANN), Random Tree (RT), Support Vector Machine (SVM), Random Tree (RTree), Artificial Neural Networks (ANN), Binary Logistic Regression, Partial Least Square Regression (PlsR), Decision Tree (DT), Convolutional Neural Network (CNN), Deep Neural Network (DNN), and the Deep Belief Network (DBF), for the diagnosis PD from speech processing. After analyzing these classifiers, they stated that the deep belief network (DBF) outperformed all other classifiers. They also stated that running deep learning techniques-architectures for medicine (in terms of i.e. early diagnosing PD) tested to be very effective and efficient [19].

There are also many studies in the literature using the Oxford Parkinson's Disease Detection Dataset and artificial intelligence techniques for the diagnosis of PD. Some of these were given as examples.

Spadoto et al. used the Optimum Path Forest (OPF) classifier and the Oxford dataset for a PD automatic diagnostic [20]. Karunanithi et al. used a fuzzy height logic method with a mathematical derivative to more accurately diagnose PD and healthy values. Using mean values and standard deviation values, they provided accurate separation of PD and healthy individuals. They used the Oxford Parkinson's Disease Data Set to test the proposed method for PD and healthy diagnosis using a fuzzy height logic method. They stated that it is a method that gives more accurate results than the current studies [21]. Revett et al. in their study, in order to determine whether features can be used to differentiate healthy individuals from those diagnosed with IPD, they used the rough set theory which is a data mining technique used in the discovery of patterns in the data. At the end of study, they said that they differentiate between IPD and healthy individuals with 100% accuracy [7]. Gill and Manuel proposed a method based on ANN and SVM to assist the specialist in the diagnosis of PD. They tested the performance of the proposed system using data from 195 examinations performed on 31 patients in the Oxford database. Their results show that an SVM has the highest accuracy rate with 93.33% [2]. Multi Layered Feedforward Neural Network model (MLFNN) with back propagation algorithm are other recommended methods for early detection and diagnosis of PD using the K-Mean Clustering algorithm [22]. In another works various data mining techniques such as Bayesian Network, Naive Bayes, J48, Sequential Minimal Optimization (SMO), and Multi-Layer Perceptron were used to develop classifier for diagnosis of Parkinson's disease. The reached experimental results at the end showed that the Multi-Layer Perceptron (MLP) have gave the highest specificity, accuracy, and also sensitivity compared to the other classifiers [23].

In his study, Zhang described the classification of PD (automatically), by using time frequency characteristics that are get by selecting features with the stacked automatic encoders (SAE) and classifying with the nearest neighbor (KNN) classifier. The reached results indicate that the related method provides better performance in the sense of the all cases tested during classification tasks and machine learning, which can classify PD to the level of competence (as comparable to doctors). Therefore, he concluded that a smartphone could potentially provide cost-effective PD diagnostic care. The article also reports the cost of uptime by giving an application on the client/server system. Both the advantages and disadvantages of the introduced tele diagnosis system are discussed [24].

5.2 Materials and Methods

In this part of the book, the diagnosis of Parkinson's disease (PD) is described using the features of speech recordings in the dataset of the Oxford Parkinson's Disease Diagnosis. In practice, Autoencoder network (AEN) was used to differentiate PD and healthy data by classifying the features in the dataset. The properties and methods of the used dataset are briefly described below. For all classification study, MATLAB r2017a software was used.

5.2.1 The Dataset of Oxford Parkinson's Disease Diagnosis

The characteristics of speech recordings in the dataset of the Oxford Parkinson's Disease Diagnosis in the UCI ML Repository [25–27] were classified and differentiated between PD and healthy individuals. Briefly, the dataset was provided Max Little, with the common works done with the National Centre for Voice and Speech (located at Denver, Colorado, USA) where the speech signals were recorded. Feature extraction methods regarding general voice disorders were published before, as the first research work-paper.

The dataset includes different biomedical voice measurements obtained from a total of 31 people including 23 with the PD. In the data set, each column corresponds to a particular voice measure. On the other hand, each row is the one of 195-voice recording from the related people. The diagnosis is made accordingly by considering the status column showing 1 for PD, and 0 for healthy person (as a classification approach over two-class decision). The dataset contains 195 entries for a total of 22 properties. These features and their definitions are shown in the context of Table 5.1 [28, 29].

Table 5.1 The definitions of features in the dataset

Feature number	Feature name	Description
1	MDVP: Fo (Hz)	Average vocal fundamental
2	MDVP: Fhi (Hz)	Maximum vocal fundamental frequency
3	MDVP: Flo (Hz)	Minimum vocal fundamental frequency
4	MDVP: Jitter (%)	Kay Pentax MDVP jitter as percentage
5	MDVP: Jitter (Abs)	Kay Pentax MDVP absolute jitter in microseconds
6	MDVP: RAP	Kay Pentax MDVP relative amplitude perturbation
7	MDVP: PPQ	Kay Pentax MDVP five-point period perturbation quotient
8	Jitter: DDP	Average absolute difference of differences between cycles, divided by the average period
9	MDVP: Shimmer	Key Pentax MDVP local shimmer
10	MDVP: Shimmer (dB)	Key Pentax MDVP local shimmer in decibels
11	Shimmer: APQ3	3 point amplitude perturbation quotient
12	Shimmer: APQ5	5 point amplitude perturbation quotient
13	MDVP: APQ	Kay Pentax MDVP eleven-point amplitude perturbation quotient
14	Shimmer: DDA	Average absolute difference between consecutive differences between the amplitude of consecutive periods
15	NHR	Noise to harmonic ratio
16	HNR	Harmonics to noise ratio
17	RPDE	Recurrence period density entropy
18	DFA	Detrended fluctuation analysis
19	Spread1	Nonlinear measure of fundamental frequency
20	Spread2	Nonlinear measure of fundamental frequency
21	D2	Pitch period entropy
22	PPE	Pitch
23	Status	Health status 1-Parkinson; 0-Healthy

5.2.2 Classification

In practice, Autoencoder network (AEN) was used to differentiate PD and healthy data by classifying the features in the dataset. The general structure of AEN is briefly explained below.

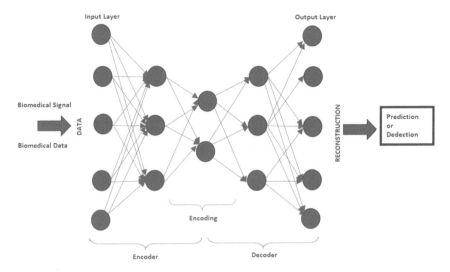

Fig. 5.1 The basic structure of an example AEN

5.2.2.1 Autoencoder Neural Network

An autoencoder network (AEN) is a feedforward neural network, which can be trained to try to copy its input(s) to the output(s). Figure 5.1 illustrates the basic structure of an example AEN.

In autoencoders (AE), the input data is converted firstly towards an abstract representation. Next, it is returned to the original format thanks to the encoder function. Furthermore, the model is trained so that the whole input is encoded into a notation, from which the input can be again reconstructed. In fact, the AE simulates something like an identity function in the context of that process. A significant advantage of AE is that it is able to obtain consistently useful properties along the propagation, and to accordingly filter useless information. In addition, efficiency of the learning process is increased because the input vector (data) is transformed into a representation at lower-dimension (during the coding process) [30].

As mentioned before, AE is a feedforward neural network that is the only hidden layer that resembles Multilayer Perseptron (MLP). The main difference between the AE and the MLP is associated with the objectives that the AE aims reconstructing the input while the MLP aims estimating the target values with the associated inputs. In a typical AE model, total number of neurons at the input layer and the output layer is same. As the first task, the AE converts the x: input vector into the h: a hidden representation, thanks to a weight matrix, let's say w. That's called as the encoding process. Following to that, the AE maps h back to its original format so that another x' with weight matrix w' is obtained. Here, the w' should be the transpose of the w. That process is the decoding. Parameter optimization is used to minimize the mean error of reconstruction between x and the x'. Here, mean square errors (MSEs) are used so that the accuracy of the measure reconstruction accuracy, as based on the assumed distribution of input properties [30, 31].

AE's strength is in the form of training for this restructuring. During reconfiguration, the activity of the hidden layer encoded only as properties from the input uses the information in h. If the model can perfectly recover the original input, then there is enough information about the input, and the learned nonlinear transformation defined by these weights and biases is a good feature extraction step. Thus, stacking of such trained coders minimizes the loss of information. At the same time, they protect abstract and immutable information in deeper properties. This is why we chose AE to gradually remove the deep properties for hyperspectral data [32].

5.2.3 Evaluating the Performance

In this study, the performance metrics of accuracy, precision, recall, f-measure, specificity, and sensitivity [33] are determined in order to evaluate the precision of the employed classification model-architecture.

Performance evaluators have important roles within the classification tasks. The most popular criteria the proportion of correct decisions taken by a classifier. Sensitivity which is also called recall, shows how much the classifier is able to recognize positive examples. Additionally, specificity is for seeing how much the classifier is good at recognizing negatives. Precision is a really positive prediction rate of positive samples. It is known that there is a decreasing hyperbolic relationship between sensitivity and precision, and one way to deal with it is using ROC charts (these graphs were for visualizing as well as selecting and organizing the classifiers by considering their performances). A ROC graph is two-dimensional, in which the FP ratio (1—specificity) is plotted over the horizontal axis and the precision is plotted over the vertical axis. Also, F-measure is the harmonic mean of sensitivity and precision [34]:

$$Accuracy = \frac{TP + TN}{TP + TN + FP + FN} \tag{5.1}$$

$$Sensitivity = \frac{TP}{TP + FN} \tag{5.2}$$

$$Specificity = \frac{TN}{FPTN + TN} \tag{5.3}$$

$$Precision = \frac{TP}{TP + FP} \tag{5.4}$$

$$Recall = Sensitivity \tag{5.5}$$

$$F\text{-measure} = 2 * \left[\frac{(Precision * Recall)}{(Precision + Recall)} \right] \quad (5.6)$$

In these Eqs. (5.1)–(5.6), TP and FP are used for indicating the number of true positive, and the number of false positive diagnosis. TN and FN are for the numbers of true negatives, and false negatives, respectively. FPTN also represents the number of false positives and it is calculated from negative samples in the findings within classification.

For the classifier, accuracy refers to the accuracy of the correct diagnosis. The sensitivity ratio indicates how accurately the classifier defines the occurrence of the target class. The specificity ratio is used to define the classifier's ability to allocate the target class. Precision is a measure of the quality of precise or accurate results. Recall, also known as true positive rate and provides the proportion of positively defined positives in a test. The F-measure is also known as the F1 score and provides a metric of the accuracy of a test. It is the weighted harmonic mean of sensitivity and recall [34–37].

5.3 Classification Application

In this chapter, it is tried to find the most suitable Autoencoder network with different experiments. The architecture of AEN is given in Fig. 5.2. As it can be observed in the figure, the AEN consists of a total of 8 stages. The first stage is an automatic identifier of hidden layer size 10 which uses a linear transfer function for the decoder. The loss function to be used for training corresponds to the mean square error function and includes L2 weight regulation and redundancy regulation. Here, the L2 weight regulator coefficient is 0.001, the coefficient for the sparsity regulation term is 4 and the sparsity ratio is 0.05. The decoder transfer function, which is the last process of the Autoencoder 1, is selected as "purelin". The scaled conjugate gradient descent algorithm is run for training the Autoencoder 1. The second stage of AEN is Features 1. Parses the features in the hidden layer that encodes Autoencoder 1 and the input matrix. The third step of AEN is Autoencoder 2 and has the same features as Autoencoder 1. It was trained using the features on the first autoencoder without scaling the data. Properties 2 extracts the properties from the hidden layer that encodes Autoencoder 2 and properties 1. The fifth stage of AEN is the SoftMax layer and is trained for classification using the 2 features of Autoencoder 2. The Softmax layer created for classification is returned as a network object. The Softmax layer is the same size as the target matrix. The loss function for the Softmax layer is the cross entropy function. In the sixth stage of AEN, the encoders and softmax layer are stacked to form the deep network Deepnet 1. In the seventh stage, the deep network is trained for the properties of sounds using input and output matrices to create Deepnet 2. Using Deepnet 1, Deepnet 2 estimates output class for input data. The maximum number of trial periods for each AEN step is 1000.

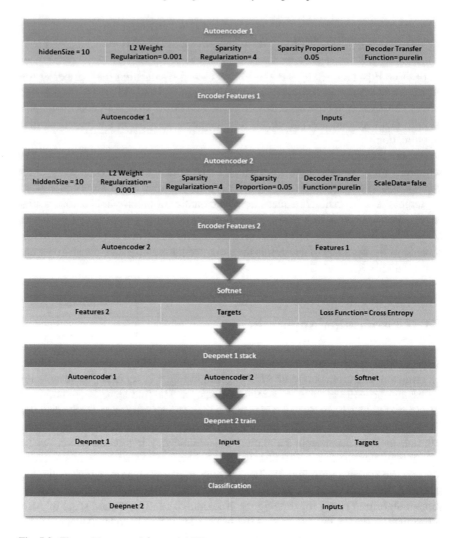

Fig. 5.2 The architecture of the used AEN

The last step predicted types for the 2 output classes such as PD or healthy for input data using Deepnet 2. This completes the classification and made prediction.

In the classification application, randomly selected 80% samples from the dataset of the Oxford Parkinson's Disease Diagnosis was used as training data whereas the remaining 20% samples was used as the test data. The classification study was repeated 20 times for randomly selected different training and test data.

5.4   Results and Discussion

In the classification application, randomly selected 80% samples from the employed dataset was used as training data and the remaining 20% samples was used as the test data. The classification study was repeated 20 times for randomly selected different training and test data. In the classification trials, the obtained performance measures were given in Table 5.2, which were the accuracy, specificity, sensitivity, precision, recall, and F-measure.

As can be seen from the table, quite high values were obtained. In order to better interpret the performance criteria of the in-classification trials, the lowest, the average and the highest values for each criterion are given in Table 5.3.

As it can be understood from the table, the lowest classification accuracy rate was 91.8%, the average classification accuracy rate was 96.1%, and the highest classification accuracy rate was 100.0%. The lowest classification sensitivity and recall rates were 95.9%, the average classification sensitivity and recall rates were 98.2%, and the highest classification sensitivity and recall rates were 100.0%. The lowest

Table 5.2 The obtained performance criterias in the classification trials

Trial no	Accuracy	Sensitivity	Specificity	Precision	Recall	F-measure
1	0.9886	0.9924	0.9767	0.9924	0.9924	0.9924
2	1	1	1	1	1	1
3	0.9423	0.9834	0.8000	0.9444	0.9835	0.9636
4	0.9231	0.9660	0.7917	0.9342	0.9660	0.9498
5	1	1	1	1	1	1
6	0.9371	0.9774	0.8095	0.9420	0.9774	0.9594
7	0.9746	0.9864	0.9375	0.9797	0.9864	0.9831
8	0.9745	0.9829	0.9487	0.9829	0.9829	0.9829
9	0.9897	0.9932	0.9792	0.9932	0.9932	0.9932
10	0.9179	0.9524	0.8125	0.9395	0.9524	0.9459
11	0.9333	0.9728	0.8125	0.9408	0.9728	0.9565
12	0.9231	0.9660	0.7916	0.9342	0.9659	0.9498
13	0.9385	0.9728	0.8333	0.9470	0.9728	0.9597
14	1	1	1	1	1	1
15	0.9641	0.9796	0.9167	0.9730	0.9796	0.9763
16	0.9538	0.9796	0.8750	0.9600	0.9796	0.9697
17	0.9231	0.9592	0.8125	0.9400	0.9592	0.9495
18	0.9436	0.9728	0.8547	0.9533	0.9728	0.9630
19	0.9949	0.9932	1	1	0.9932	0.9966
20	1	1	1	1	1	1
Mean	0.9611	0.9815	0.8978	0.9678	0.9815	0.9745

Table 5.3 The lowest, the average and the highest values of performance criterias

Criteria	Lowest	Average	Highest
Accuracy	0.9179	0.9611	1
Sensitivity	0.9592	0.9815	1
Specificity	0.7916	0.8978	1
Precision	0.9342	0.9678	1
Recall	0.9592	0.9815	1
F-measure	0.9459	0.9745	1

classification specificity rate was 79.2%, the average classification specificity rate was 89.8%, and the highest classification specificity rate was 100.0%. The lowest classification precision rate was 93.4%, the average classification precision rate was 96.8%, and the highest classification precision rate was 100.0%. The lowest classification F-measure rate was 94.6%, the average classification F-measure rate was 97.5%, and the highest classification accuracy rate was 100.0%.

Classification studies for the Oxford Parkinson's dataset with AEN have high accuracy, sensitivity and specificity rates. The developed method for Oxford Parkinson's data, achieving an average overall accuracy of 96.1%, has the very high performance. In the classification study for PD diagnosis, the obtained confusion matrices in the overall, training, and test stages are given in Figs. 5.3, 5.4, 5.5, 5.6, 5.7, 5.8, 5.9, 5.10 and 5.11. Figures 5.3, 5.4 and 5.5 represent the confusion matrices in which the lowest accuracy rate is obtained. Figures 5.6, 5.7 and 5.8 show the

Fig. 5.3 The confusion matrices for the lowest accuracy rate—overall

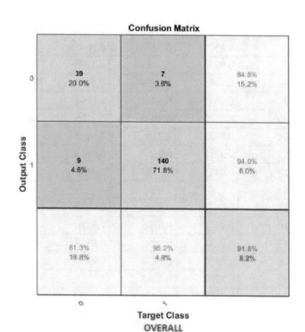

Fig. 5.4 The confusion
matrices for the lowest
accuracy rate—training

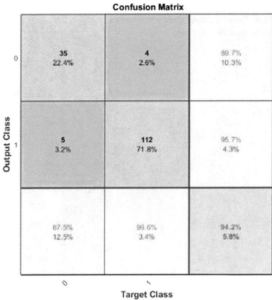

Fig. 5.5 The confusion
matrices for the lowest
accuracy rate—test

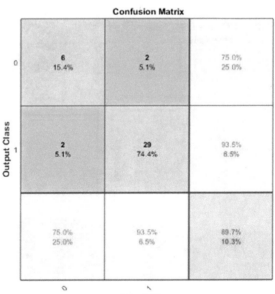

Fig. 5.6 The confusion
matrices for the average
accuracy rate—overall

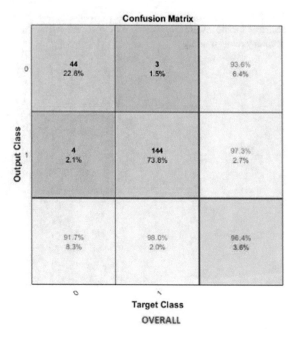

Fig. 5.7 The confusion
matrices for the average
accuracy rate—training

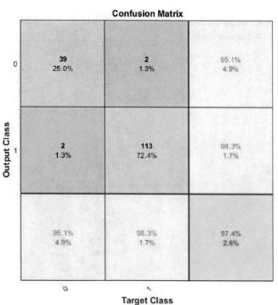

Fig. 5.8 The confusion
matrices for the average
accuracy rate—test

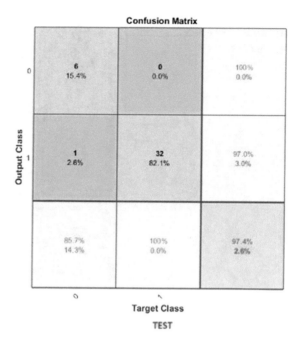

Fig. 5.9 The confusion
matrices for the highest
accuracy rate—overall

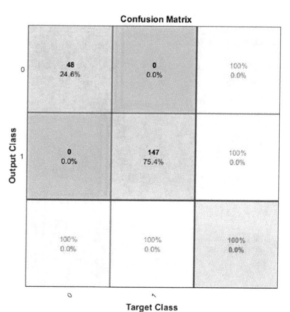

Fig. 5.10 The confusion matrices for the highest accuracy rate—training

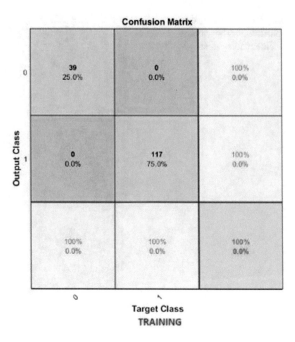

Fig. 5.11 The confusion matrices for the highest accuracy rate—test

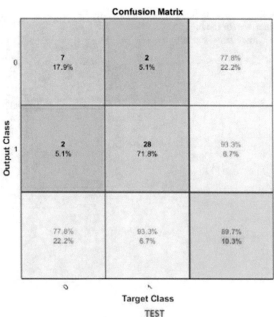

confusion matrices closest to the average accuracy rate. Figures 5.9, 5.10 and 5.11 represent the confusion matrices in which the highest accuracy rate is obtained.

The obtained high sensitivity shows that the developed model accurately defines the formation of the target class. The obtained high specificity ratio shows that the developed model has a very high ability to allocate the target class. F-measure is the harmonic mean of the classifier and its recall. In most cases, there is a balance between precision and recall. If you optimize the classifier to increase one and remove the other, the harmonic average decreases rapidly. However, when both sensitivity and recall are equal, it is the largest. If the F-measure is very high, the classifier is in very good condition.

Developed for PD diagnosis and applied with Oxford Parkinson's diagnostic data set, the obtained results in the classification study with AEN, we can say that AENs are ideal for the diagnosis of disease from a big dataset, and they work very effectively and efficiently.

5.5 Summary

Parkinson's disease (PD) is a degenerative disease in the context of the central nervous system. As following the Alzheimer's disease, PD is known among critical common neurodegenerative diseases. The number of people with PD worldwide is quite high and is rapidly increasing. It is stated that the number of PD patients will be doubled by 2030. Early diagnosis of PD disease can also reduce symptoms. Significant symptoms of PD are tremor, stiffness, slow motion, motor symptom asymmetry and impaired posture.

Recent research has reported that speech difficulties observed around the 90% of PD cases can be a remarkable sign for detecting healthy and PD patients, even in the early stages of the disease [7]. Speech disorders in PD patients can be broadly classified as dysphonia and dysarthria. Dysphonia is a deterioration in speech production as it may be showing increase according to the disease progression. Dysarthria reflects that it cannot be jointed properly. Vocal pathology is caused by dysfunction of the laryngeal, articulator and respiratory muscles. Some studies have classified the general effects of speech disorder as wind, tremendous, treble, monotonous and muffled. Sound analysis techniques, such as spectrograms and electroglottographic (EGG) recordings of images of voice samples, can be used to identify disruptions in PD patients.

In this section, the diagnosis of PD with deep learning by using the data obtained from Oxford Parkinson Diagnostic Data is investigated and the performance of deep learning is discussed. The diagnosis of Parkinson's disease (PD) is described using the features of speech recordings in the dataset of the Oxford Parkinson's Disease Diagnosis. In practice, Autoencoder network (AEN) was used to differentiate PD and healthy individual data by classifying the features in the dataset. The properties and methods of the dataset and the used methods were briefly described. For all classification study, MATLAB r2017a software was used.

Classification studies for the Oxford Parkinson's dataset with AEN have high accuracy, sensitivity and specificity rates. The developed method for Oxford Parkinson's data, achieving an average overall accuracy of 96.1%, has the very high performance.

The obtained high sensitivity explains us that the developed model accurately defines the formation of the target class. The obtained high specificity ratio points that the developed model has a very high ability to allocate the target class. F-measure is the harmonic mean of the classifier and its recall. In most cases, there is a balance between precision and recall. If you optimize the classifier to increase one and remove the other, the harmonic average decreases rapidly. However, when both sensitivity and recall are equal, it is the largest. If the F-measure is very high, the classifier is in very good condition.

Developed for PD diagnosis and applied with Oxford Parkinson's diagnostic data set, the obtained results in the classification study with AEN, we can say that AENs are ideal for the diagnosis of disease from a big dataset, and they work very effectively and efficiently.

As deep learning seems like a solution with complex features to be understood, it is actually a revolutionary tool for providing decision support tools, which are easier to use when compared with traditional machine learning solutions or hybrid systems developed with them. The next chapter aims to show that it is possible to do that by considering heart diseases. As different from Parkinson's, that was done that time by working on raw data, as explained in Chap. 6.

5.6 Further Learning

In order to investigate details regarding the characteristics of AE techniques and methods, [38–45] can be seen.

The articles in [46–48] can be examined to see the applications and performances of AEN in different databases.

The use of Autoencoder in a speech enhancement noise classification [49] could be seen. Also, to see the performance of Autoencoder in a speech and an audio recognition [45, 50, 51] can be read.

In a mobile application for the diagnosis of Parkinson's disease, [24] can be examined to see details of the use of two separate databases, different for education and different for classification.

In order to see different methods in PD diagnosis, a hybrid intelligent system that predicts PD progression using noise reduction, clustering and prediction methods can be examined [52]. In this study, Principal Component Analysis (PCA) and Expectation Maximization (EM) were used to address the multiple-co-linearity problems in the experimental data sets and to cluster the data. Adaptive Neuro-Fuzzy Inference System (ANFIS) and then Support Vector Regression (SVR) were applied to predict PD progression. Experimental results on public Parkinson's datasets have been suggested to significantly improve the accuracy of predicting PD progression of the proposed method. In the hybrid intelligent system, instead of SVR, AEN or another deep learning method can be considered. Also, to see a different approach for PD diagnosis [1] might be read.

References

1. Z. Cai, J. Gu, C. Wen, D. Zhao, C. Huang, H. Huang, C. Tong, J. Li, H. Chen, An intelligent Parkinson's disease diagnostic system based on a chaotic bacterial foraging optimization enhanced fuzzy KNN approach. Comput. Math. Methods Med. **2018**, 24 (2018)
2. D. Gil, D.J. Manuel, Diagnosing Parkinson by using artificial neural networks and support vector machines. Glob. J. Comput. Sci. Technol. **9**(4), 63–71 (2009)
3. A. Elbaz, J.H. Bower, D.M. Maraganore, S.K. McDonnell, B.J. Peterson, J.E. Ahlskog, D.J. Schaid, W.A. Rocca, Risk tables for Parkinsonism and Parkinson's disease. J. Clin. Epidemiol. **55**(1), 25–31 (2002)
4. E. Dorsey, R. Constantinescu, J.P. Thompson, K.M. Biglan, R.G. Holloway, K. Kieburtz, F.J. Marshall, B.M. Ravina, G. Schifitto, A. Siderowf, C.M. Tanner, Projected number of people with Parkinson disease in the most populous nations, 2005 through 2030. Neurology **68**(5), 384–386 (2007)
5. R.G. Ramani, G. Sivagami, Parkinson disease classification using data mining algorithms. Int. J. Comput. Appl. **32**(9), 17–22 (2011)
6. Parkinson's Disease Foundation, https://www.parkinson.org/. Last access 04 Jan 2020
7. K. Revett, F. Gorunescu, A.B.M. Salem, Feature selection in Parkinson's disease: a rough sets approach, in *2009 International Multiconference on Computer Science and Information Technology* (IEEE, 2009), pp. 425–428
8. S.S. Rao, L.A. Hofmann, A. Shakil, Parkinson's disease: diagnosis and treatment. Am. Fam. Phys. **74**(12), 2046–2054 (2006)
9. M. Ene, Neural network-based approach to discriminate healthy people from those with Parkinson's disease. Ann. Univ. Craiova Math. Comput. Sci. Ser. **35**, 112–116 (2008)
10. M. Gil-Martín, J.M. Montero, R. San-Segundo, Parkinson's disease detection from drawing movements using convolutional neural networks. Electronics **8**(8), 907 (2019)
11. C.R. Pereira, S.A. Weber, C. Hook, G.H. Rosa, J.P. Papa, Deep learning-aided Parkinson's disease diagnosis from handwritten dynamics, in *2016 29th SIBGRAPI Conference on Graphics, Patterns and Images (SIBGRAPI)* (IEEE, 2016), pp. 340–346
12. S.L. Oh, Y. Hagiwara, U. Raghavendra, R. Yuvaraj, N. Arunkumar, M. Murugappan, Acharya, U.R. Murugappan, A deep learning approach for Parkinson's disease diagnosis from EEG signals. Neural Comput. Appl. 1–7 (2018)
13. H. Choi, S. Ha, H.J. Im, S.H. Paek, D.S. Lee, Refining diagnosis of Parkinson's disease with deep learning-based interpretation of dopamine transporter imaging. Neuroimage Clin. **16**, 586–594 (2017)
14. B.M. Eskofier, S.I. Lee, J.F. Daneault, F.N. Golabchi, G. Ferreira-Carvalho, G. Vergara-Diaz, S. Sapienza, G. Costante, J. Klucken, T. Kautz, P. Bonato, Recent machine learning advancements in sensor-based mobility analysis: deep learning for Parkinson's disease assessment, in *2016 38th Annual International Conference of the IEEE Engineering in Medicine and Biology Society (EMBC)* (IEEE, 2016), pp. 655–658
15. S. Sivaranjini, C.M. Sujatha, Deep learning based diagnosis of Parkinson's disease using convolutional neural network. Multimed. Tools Appl. 1–13 (2019)
16. S. Shinde, S. Prasad, Y. Saboo, R. Kaushick, J. Saini, P.K. Pal, M. Ingalhalikar, Predictive markers for Parkinson's disease using deep neural nets on neuromelanin sensitive MRI. Neuroimage Clin. **22**, 101748 (2019)

17. A. Ortiz, J. Munilla, M. Martínez, J.M. Gorriz, J. Ramírez, D. Salas-Gonzalez, Parkinson's disease detection using isosurfaces-based features and convolutional neural networks. Front. Neuroinf. **13**, 48 (2019)
18. S. Grover, S. Bhartia, A. Yadav, K.R. Seeja, Predicting severity of Parkinson's disease using deep learning. Proc. Comput. Sci. **132**, 1788–1794 (2018)
19. S. Muthumanickam, J. Gayathri, Daphne J. Eunice, Parkinson's disease detection and classification using machine learning and deep learning algorithms—a survey. Int. J. Eng. Sci. Invent. (IJESI) **7**(5), 56–63 (2018)
20. A.A. Spadoto, R.C. Guido, F.L. Carnevali, A.F. Pagnin, A.X. Falcão, J.P. Papa, Improving Parkinson's disease identification through evolutionary-based feature selection, in *2011 Annual International Conference of the IEEE Engineering in Medicine and Biology Society* (IEEE, 2011), pp. 7857–7860
21. D. Karunanithi, P. Rodrigues, Diagnosis of Parkinson's disease using fuzzy height. Int. J. Pure Appl. Math. **118**(20), 4497–4501 (2018)
22. R.F. Olanrewaju, N.S. Sahari, A.A. Musa, N. Hakiem, Application of neural networks in early detection and diagnosis of Parkinson's disease, in *2014 International Conference on Cyber and IT Service Management* (*CITSM*) (IEEE, 2014), pp. 78–82
23. P. Durga, V.S. Jebakumari, D. Shanthi, Diagnosis and classification of Parkinsons disease using data mining techniques. Int. J. Adv. Res. Trends Eng. Technol. **3**, 86–90 (2016)
24. Y.N. Zhang, Can a smartphone diagnose parkinson disease? A deep neural network method and telediagnosis system implementation, in *Parkinson's Disease* (2017)
25. M.A. Little, P.E. McSharry, S.J. Roberts, D.A. Costello, I.M. Moroz, Exploiting nonlinear recurrence and fractal scaling properties for voice disorder detection. Biomed. Eng. Online **6**(1), 23 (2007)
26. M. Little, P. McSharry, E. Hunter, J. Spielman, L. Ramig, Suitability of dysphonia measurements for telemonitoring of Parkinson's disease. Nat. Preced. 1 (2008)
27. Oxford Parkinson's Disease Detection Dataset, https://archive.ics.uci.edu/ml/datasets/parkinsons. Last access 09 Jan 2020
28. R. Geetha Ramani, G. Sivagami, Parkinson disease classification using data mining algorithms. Int. J. Comput. Appl. **32**(9) (2011) (0975-8887)
29. X. Wang, Data mining analysis of the Parkinson's disease. Mathematics Theses, Georgia State University, 17 Feb 2014
30. W. Liu, Z. Wang, X. Liu, N. Zeng, Y. Liu, F.E. Alsaadi, A survey of deep neural network architectures and their applications. Neurocomputing **234**, 11–26 (2017)
31. Y. Bengio, P. Lamblin, D. Popovici, H. Larochelle, Greedy layer-wise training of deep networks. Adv. Neural. Inf. Process. Syst. **19**, 153–160 (2007)
32. Y. Chen, Z. Lin, X. Zhao, G. Wang, Y. Gu, Deep learning-based classification of hyperspectral data. IEEE J. Sel. Top. Appl. Earth Observ. Rem. Sens. **7**(6), 2094–2107 (2014)
33. W. Zhang, J. Han, S. Deng, Heart sound classification based on scaled spectrogram and tensor decomposition. Biomed. Signal Process. Control **32**, 20–28 (2017)
34. R.P. Espíndola, N.F.F. Ebecken, On extending F-measure and G-mean metrics to multi-class problems. WIT Trans. Inf. Commun. Technol. 35
35. O. Deperlioglu, Classification of phonocardiograms with convolutional neural networks. BRAIN Broad Res. Artif. Intell. Neurosci. **9**(2), 23–33 (2018)
36. D.J. Hemanth, O. Deperlioglu, U. Kose, An enhanced diabetic retinopathy detection and classification approach using deep convolutional neural network. Neural Comput. Appl. **32**, 1–15 (2020)
37. Q.-A. Mubarak, M.U. Akram, A. Shaukat, F. Hussain, S.G. Khawaja, W.H. Butt, Analysis of PCG signals using quality assessment and homomorphic filters for localization and classification of heart sounds. Comput. Methods Program. Biomed. (2018). https://doi.org/10.1016/j.cmpb.2018.07.006
38. L. Deng, D. Yu, Deep learning: methods and applications. Found. Trends Sig. Process. **7**(3–4), 197–387 (2014)
39. I. Goodfellow, Y. Bengio, A. Courville, in *Deep Learning* (MIT Press, 2016)

40. Y. LeCun, Y. Bengio, G. Hinton, Deep learning. Nature **521**(7553), 436–444 (2015)
41. Deep Learning Tutorial, in *Release 0.1, LISA Lab.* University of Montreal, Sept 2015
42. A. Zhang, Z.C. Lipton, M. Li, A.J. Smola, Dive into deep learning, in *Unpublished Draft.* Retrieved, Mar 2019, p. 319
43. P. Baldi, Autoencoders, unsupervised learning, and deep architectures, in *Proceedings of ICML Workshop on Unsupervised and Transfer Learning*, June 2012, pp. 37–49
44. Q.V. Le, A tutorial on deep learning part 2: autoencoders, convolutional neural networks and recurrent neural networks. Google Brain 1–20 (2015)
45. S. Amiriparian, M. Freitag, N. Cummins, B. Schuller, Sequence to sequence autoencoders for unsupervised representation learning from audio, in *Proceedings of the DCASE 2017 Workshop*, Nov 2017
46. O. Deperlioglu, Classification of segmented heart sounds with autoencoder neural networks, in *VIII. International Multidisciplinary Congress of Eurasia* (*IMCOFE'2019*) (Antalya, 2019), 24–26 Apr 2019, pp. 122–128. ISBN: 978-605-68882-6-7
47. O. Deperlioglu, Hepatitis disease diagnosis with deep neural networks, in *International 4th European Conference on Science, Art & Culture* (*ECSAC'2019*) (Antalya, 2019), 18–21 Apr 2019, pp. 467–473. ISBN: 978-605-7809-73-5
48. O. Deperlioglu, Using autoencoder deep neural networks for diagnosis of breast cancer, in *International 4th European Conference on Science, Art & Culture* (*ECSAC'2019*) (Antalya, 2019), 18–21 Apr 2019, pp. 475–481. ISBN: 978-605-7809-73-5
49. B. Xia, C. Bao, Wiener filtering based speech enhancement with weighted denoising auto-encoder and noise classification. Speech Commun. **60**, 13–29 (2014)
50. K. Noda, Y. Yamaguchi, K. Nakadai, H.G. Okuno, T. Ogata, Audio-visual speech recognition using deep learning. Appl. Intell. **42**(4), 722–737 (2015)
51. R.G. Malkin, A. Waibel, Classifying user environment for mobile applications using linear autoencoding of ambient audio, in *Proceedings* (*ICASSP'05*). *IEEE International Conference on Acoustics, Speech, and Signal Processing, 2005*, vol. 5 (IEEE, 2005), pp v–509
52. M. Nilashi, O. Ibrahim, A. Ahani, Accuracy improvement for predicting Parkinson's disease progression. Sci. Rep. **6**, 34181 (2016)

Chapter 6
A Practical Method for Early Diagnosis of Heart Diseases via Deep Neural Network

Nowadays, the majority of human deaths are from heart diseases. For this reason, many studies have been done to improve the early diagnosis of heart diseases and to reduce deaths. These studies are mostly aimed at developing computer-aided diagnostic systems using the developing technology. Some computer-aided systems are clinical decision support systems that are developed to more easily detect heart disease than heart sounds or related data. These systems are software used in the automatic diagnosis of heart diseases, which are generally based on the classification of data. Most of the studies used to diagnose heart diseases are for increasing the success of classification [1, 2].

Bathia and colleagues have developed a decision-making support system to classify heart diseases using a support vector machine and an integer-value-coded genetic algorithm. In this study, the genetic algorithm is used to maximize the performance of the simple support vector machine, select the relevant properties, and delete the unnecessary ones [3]. Parthibane and Subramanian suggested a method based on co-operative neuro-fuzzy inference (CANFIS) for predicting heart disease. This CANFIS model combined the qualitative approach to fuzzy logic integrated with the genetic algorithm to diagnose the capabilities of the neural network and then the presence of the disease [4].

There is a lot of data in health systems. However, effective analysis tools are required to explore the hidden relationships and trends in the data. For this purpose, the discovery of information and the use of data mining are the most important topics in scientific studies. Researchers have long used statistical and also data mining techniques for making results better for data analysis in large data sets. Diagnosis of disease is one of the widely-done applications in which data mining techniques have achieved successful results. Ahmed and Hannan in their research, they have experimented to find heart diseases with data mining, Support Vector Machine, Genetic Algorithm, coarse set theory, merger rules, and Artificial Neural Networks. They have found that the decision tree and SVM are the most effective for heart disease. Therefore, they stated that data mining can help to identify or predict high or low risk

U. Kose et al., *Deep Learning for Medical Decision Support Systems*, Studies in Computational Intelligence 909, https://doi.org/10.1007/978-981-15-6325-6_6

heart diseases [5]. Another data mining study analyzed prediction systems for Heart disease using more input characteristics. The data mining classification techniques such as Naive Bayes, Decision Trees, and also Artificial Neural Networks are evaluated over Heart disease database. General performance of these related techniques is compared and, respectively, Artificial Neural Networks, Decision Trees, and Naive Bayes' classification accuracy rates were high [6]. As we have seen, Artificial Neural Network has been widely used for the diagnosing heart diseases. The related work of Das et al. [7] and the work by Deperlioglu are also examples of recent studies [2].

Recently, deep learning methods have also been used to classify heart sounds. For example, Potes and colleagues have proposed a method based on a classifier group that combines the outputs of AdaBoost and Convolutional Neural Network (CNN) for performing classification regarding abnormal/normal heart sounds [8]. Rubin et al. have proposed an automatic heart sound classification algorithm that allows time-frequency heat map indications to be combined with a CNN [9]. Deperlioglu in his studies used CNN to classify phonocardiograms segmented and non-segmented in their study [10, 11].

As can be seen from the above examples, complex mixed methods are generally employed in diagnosing heart disease in order to increase classification success. In this chapter, use of a deep learning method to increase the success of the diagnosis of heart diseases (without dealing with more complicated methods or algorithms) was examined. The chapter briefly will focus on the detection of heart diseases using the Cleveland Heart Disease data set and Autoencoder Neural Networks (AEN). In addition, the chapter is for showing that the classification success can be increased easily by using (AEN) without any feature selection process or mixed methods.

6.1 Fundamentals

In this chapter, it was explained that the determination of cardiac diseases using the Cleveland Heart Disease data set and AEN can be easily classified without any feature selection process or mixed methods. Materials and methods used for the study are given in detail below.

6.1.1 Cleveland Heart Disease Data Set

In order to test proposed method, the Cleveland Heart Database taken from UCI learning dataset repository was used [12–15]. The Cleveland Heart Disease database consists of 303 records with 13 attributes. These attributes are given in Table 6.1.

Almost all studies conducted for the diagnosis of heart disease with this database have used the above-mentioned 13 properties as input [6]. The data in the data set consisted of 5 output classes, 1, 2, 3, 4 indicating the presence of heart disease, and 0 indicating the absence.

Table 6.1 Definition of 13 input attributes

No.	Attribute	Definition	Value(s)
1	Age	Age (as year)	Real (number)
2	Sex	Female or Male	0 = female/1 = male
3	CP	Type of chest pain	4 = asymptomatic 3 = non-agina pain 2 = typical type agina 1 = typical type 1
4	Thestbps	Pressure of resting blood	Real (number) value/mm hg
5	Chol	Serum cholesterol	Real (number) value/mm/dl
6	Restecg	Electrographic results in the context of resting	0 = normal 1 = having_ST_T wave abnormal 2 = left ventricular hypertrophy
7	Fbs	Sugar in fasting blood	$1 \geq 120$ mg/dl $0 \leq 120$ mg/dl
8	Thalach	Max. value of the heart rate	Real (number) value
9	Exang	Exercise induced agina	0 = no 1 = yes
10	Oldpeak	ST depression state as induced by exercise relative to rest	Real (number) value
11	Solpe	Slope of the peak exercise ST segment	3 = downsloping 2 = flat 1 = unsloping
12	CA	As colored by flour sopy, number of major vessels	value within 0-3
13	Thal	Type of defect	7 = reversible defect 6 = fixed 3 = normal

6.1.2 Autoencoder Neural Network

Autoencoder neural networks were first introduced by Hinton and Salakhutdinov in 2006 [16]. Basically, it can be thought of as forward-feed neural networks trained to be reliable replicates of inputs. But the network model is structured such that the intermediate layers employ less neurons than the upper and lower level layers. Therefore, the network may be considered as an encoder-decoder pair associated with the least number of neurons containing the encoded representation of the inputs. Because each layer only depends on the values of the previous layer, the knowledge of the encoding is sufficient to calculate the respective reconstruction [17]. Commonly, auto-coding networks are defined by setting the number of nodes in each layer. Figure 6.1 shows the model-architecture of an Autencoder network. The successive node layers detect patterns in the input data and use them to generate an encoded representation of the data. It receives the corresponding decoder encodings and attempts to reconfigure the original entries. The network training algorithm involves adjusting the behavior of each node to bring the configurations closer to the data. Networks can be defined

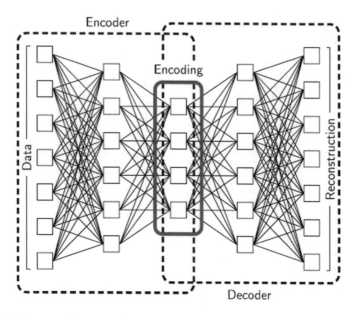

Fig. 6.1 Architecture of an automatic encoder network [17]

by the number of nodes in each layer. For example, the network shown in Fig. 6.1 has five node layers interconnected by four neuronal layers and is 7-6-4-6-7 Autencoder [17].

Automatic coders belong to a class-learning algorithm known as unsupervised learning, and unchecked learning algorithms do not need tagged information for data [18].

6.1.3   Performance Evaluation

The accuracy, sensitivity and specificity are commonly used performance measures in medical classification studies. These measures were used to assess the precision of the proposed method. They are calculated as the following:

$$Ac = \frac{T_P}{T_P + F_P} \tag{6.1}$$

$$Se = \frac{T_P}{T_P + F_N} \tag{6.2}$$

$$Sp = \frac{T_N}{F_{PTN} + T_N} \tag{6.3}$$

In the equations, T_P and F_P represents the numbers respectively for true positives and false positives. On the other hand, T_N and F_N are respectively for the numbers of true negatives, and false negatives. F_{PTN} also represents the number of false positives and it is calculated from negative samples in the results of classification.

The precision of the classifier's ability to diagnose correctly is determined by the ratio of accuracy. The extent to which the model correctly defines the formation of the target class is defined by the rate of Sensitivity. The extent of the model's target class separation capability is defined by the rate of Specificity [10].

6.2 Early Diagnosis of Heart Diseases

At the end of a large number of trials with the Cleveland Heart Database data set, parameters of AEN were obtained. The structure and details of AEN, which consists of 8 stages in total, are given in Fig. 6.2.

In the classification study with AEN, there are 24 hidden layers in the network. In the coding stage, the scale was used as a scale algorithm and the function of the cross-entropy cost function was used. In the decoding phase, Levenberg-Marquardt algorithm and mean quadratic error method were used.

With the obtained AEN, 80% of the datasets and 20% of the data were classified as test data. Randomly selected, different training and test data and classification process was repeated 20 times. The rates for accuracy, sensitivity, and specificity (as obtained in these studies) were averaged. As a result of the experiments, the confusion matrices for the lowest and highest accuracy rates are given in Figs. 6.3, and 6.4, respectively.

At the end of 20 trials, the mean accuracy rate was 99.13%, sensitivity was 97.90%, and specificity was 97.95%.

In order to evaluate the performance of the proposed method was compared with the results of previous studies which used the same data set. These are: (1) Deperlioglu used artificial neural networks (ANN) with Bayesian regulation algorithm [1]. (2) Bathia and others used genetic algorithms (GA) for selection of features and simple support vector machine (SSVM) for classification [3]. (3) Kahramanli and Allahverdi used a hybrid method that includes artificial neural network (ANN) and fuzzy neural network (FNN) [21]. (4) Anooj used weighted fuzzy rules (WFR). (5) Das et al. used A neural networks ensemble method (ANN) [7]. (6) Setiawan et al. used fuzzy decision support system (FDSS) with rules extraction method based on Rough Set Theory [20]. (7)–(9) They also used multi-layer perceptron ANN (MLP ANN), k-Nearest Neighbor (k-NN), C4.5 and RIPPER method for comparison [20]. (10) Details are given in Table 6.2. The highest values in the table are given as bold.

As it can be understood from Table 6.2, the proposed method gives better results than many single or hybrid methods. The accuracy rate of 99.13% indicates that the accuracy of the correct diagnostic capability of the classifier is high. The sensitivity ratio in 97.90% indicates that the model has a high degree of accurate determination

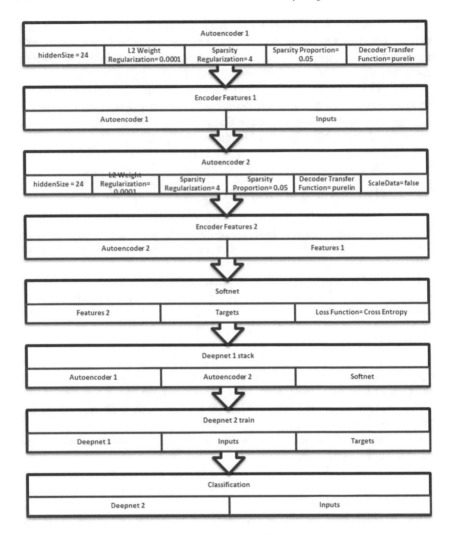

Fig. 6.2 The structure and details of autoencoder neural network

of the formation of the target class. The specificity ratio of 97.95% indicates that the model has a broad scope of target class separation capability.

6.3   Results and Discussion

Many biomedical decision support systems have been developed to reduce early death from heart disease by developing early diagnosis. The researchers have tried to

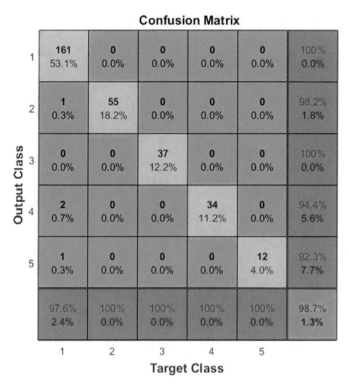

Fig. 6.3 The confusion matrices for the lowest accuracy rates

increase the efficiency with mixed methods by using different methods such as optimization methods together with classification techniques. In this study, it is explained that the accuracy of classification can be increased by using autoencoder neural network from deep neural networks without using mixed methods or feature selection with different optimization methods. For this purpose, the Cleveland Heart Disease data set, which is widely used in medical databases in the University of California Irvine (UCI) machine learning laboratory, was used. The obtained accuracy, sensitivity and specificity values by the proposed method show that the method has high performance. Thus, with much less workload, heart diseases can be diagnosed in a shorter time.

6.4 Summary

As the majority of human deaths are from heart diseases, many alternative studies have been done to improve the early diagnosis of heart dis-eases and to reduce deaths. These studies are mostly aimed at developing computer-aided diagnostic systems

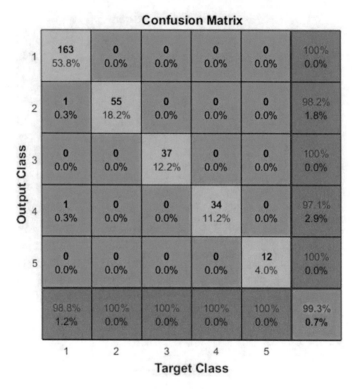

Fig. 6.4 The confusion matrices for the highest accuracy rates

using the developing technology. Some computer-aided systems are clinical decision support systems that are developed to more easily detect heart disease than heart sounds or related data. These systems are software used in the automatic diagnosis of heart diseases, which are generally based on the classification of data. At this point, deep learning techniques took the success levels to higher values thanks to their in-depth analyze and diagnosis potentials.

In this chapter, a classification study with AEN was introduced accordingly, as an easy-to-use tool for diagnosing heart diseases. As structured over 24 hidden layers form in the network, the scale was used as a scale algorithm and the function of the cross-entropy cost function was used for effective training. In the decoding phase, Levenberg-Marquardt algorithm and mean quadratic error method were used, too. The AEN was trained by 80% of the datasets and 20% of the data as testing, through randomly selected, different training and test data and classification process as repeated 20 times. The mean accuracy rate has been 99.13% while sensitivity is 97.90%, and the specificity is 97.95%. The AEN solution here was also compared with the literature and it was seen that it gives better results than many single or hybrid methods. The accuracy rate of 99.13% by the AEN indicates that the accuracy of the correct diagnostic capability of the classifier is high. With the sensitivity

Table 6.2 The comparison data of the previous studies which used the same data set

Order of study	Author	Method	Accuracy (%)	Sensitivity (%)	Specificity (%)
1	This study	AEN	**99.13**	**97.90**	**97.95**
2	Deperlioglu [1]	ANN	85.8	86.7	86.7
3	Bhatia et al. [3]	GA + SSVM	86.50	86.3	88.50
4	Kahramanli [5]	ANN + FNN	87.40	93	78.5
5	Anooj [19]	WFR	62.35	76.59	44.73
6	Das et al. [7]	ANN	89.01	80.95	95.91
7	Setiawan [20]	FDSS	81.00	83.00	85.00
8	Setiawan [20]	MLP-ANN	81.00	77.85	85.00
9	Setiawan [20]	k-NN	81.00	84.00	79.00
10	Setiawan [20]	C4.5	82.00	79.00	85.00
11	Setiawan [20]	RIPPER	83.00	82.00	84.00

ratio in 97.90%, it also has a high degree of accurate determination of the formation of the target class and it also has a broad scope of target class separation capability, considering the specificity ratio of 97.95%.

It was seen that it is possible to form an easy-to-use and even easy-to-build diagnosis model with deep learning, without needing for any complex hybrid structure or detailed processes of pre-processing and classification. Here, an example of using AEN for that purpose was shown.

Since deep learning can itself effective enough to solve target medical problems, it can be still open to develop hybrid solutions because some problems may require more advanced collaborations of different techniques. As similar to the traditional machine learning techniques, it is always possible to form a strong relation between swarm intelligence and deep learning. So, the next Chap. 7 provides an example approach for ensuring a multi-disease diagnosis system.

6.5 Further Learning

For more learning about remarkable applications of artificial intelligence for heart disease diagnosis, the readers are referred to [22–30].

In the literature, it is also possible to see use of alternative deep learning techniques for heart disease diagnosis. For some very recent works in this manner, readers can read [31–37].

As also heart attack has a critical place among all heart diseases, some of additional remarkable research works of artificial intelligence (machine/deep learning) can be read from [38–43].

References

1. O. Deperlioglu, The effects of different training algorithms on the classification of medical databases using artificial neural networks, in *European Conference on Science, Art & Culture ECSAC* (2018)
2. Ömer Deperlioğlu, Classification of segmented heart sounds with Artificial Neural Networks. Int. J. Appl. Math. Electr. Comput. **6**(4), 39–44 (2018)
3. S. Bhatia, P. Prakash, G.N. Pillai, SVM based decision support system for heart disease classification with integer-coded genetic algorithm to select critical features, in *Proceedings of the World Congress on Engineering and Computer Science* (2008)
4. L. Parthiban, R. Subramanian, Intelligent heart disease prediction system using CANFIS and genetic algorithm. Int. J. Biol. Biomed. Med. Sci. **3**(3) (2008)
5. A. Ahmed, S.A. Hannan, Data mining techniques to find out heart diseases: an overview. Int. J. Innov. Technol. Explor. Eng. (IJITEE), **1**(4) (2012). ISSN 2278-3075
6. C.S. Dangare, S. Apte Sulabha, Improved study of heart disease prediction system using data mining classification techniques, Int. J. Comput. Appl. **47**(10), 44–48 (2012)
7. Resul Das, Ibrahim Turkoglu, Abdulkadir Sengur, Effective diagnosis of heart disease through neural networks ensembles. Expert Syst. Appl. **36**(4), 7675–7680 (2009)
8. C. Potes, S. Parvaneh, A. Rahman, B. Conroy, Ensemble of feature-based and deep learning-based classifiers for detection of abnormal heart sounds. https://arxiv.org/pdf/1707.04642.pdf. 2017
9. J. Rubin, R. Abreu, A. Ganguli, S. Nelaturi, I. Matei, K. Sricharan, recognizing abnormal heart sounds using deep learning. https://physionet.org/challenge/2016/papers/potes.pdf (2017)
10. O. Deperlioglu, Classification of phonocardiograms by convolutional neural networks, BRAIN. Broad Res. Artif. Intell. Neurosci. **9**(2) (2018)
11. O. Deperlioglu, Classification of phonocardiograms by convolutional neural networks, BRAIN. Broad Res. Artif. Intell. Neurosci. **10**(1) (2019)
12. Cleveland heart disease data set. http://archive.ics.uci.edu/ml/datasets/Heart+Disease. Last Accessed 10 Jan 2019
13. Robert Detrano et al., International application of a new probability algorithm for the diagnosis of coronary artery disease. Am. J. Cardiol. **64**(5), 304–310 (1989)
14. D. Aha, D. Kibler, Instance-based prediction of heart-disease presence with the Cleveland database. Univ. Calif. **3**(1), 3–2 (1988)
15. John H. Gennari, Pat Langley, Doug Fisher, Models of incremental concept formation. Artif. Intell. **40**(1-3), 11–61 (1989)
16. G. Hinton, R. Salakhutdinov, Reducing the dimensionality of data with neural networks. Science **313**, 504–507 (2006)
17. Andrew P. Valentine, Trampert Jeannot, Data space reduction, quality assessment and searching of seismograms: autoencoder networks for waveform data. Geophys. J. Int. **189**(2), 1183–1202 (2012)
18. Q.V. Le, A tutorial on deep learning part 2: autoencoders, convolutional neural networks and recurrent neural networks. Google Brain 1–20 (2015)

19. P.K. Anooj, Clinical decision support system: Risk level prediction of heart disease using weighted fuzzy rules. J. King Saud Univ.-Comput. Inf. Sci. **24**(1), 27–40 (2012)
20. N.A. Setiawan, P.A. Venkatachalam, A.F.M. Hani, Diagnosis of coronary artery disease using artificial intelligence based decision support system, in *Proceedings of the International Conference on Man-Machine Systems (ICoMMS)* (Batu Ferringhi, Penang. 2009)
21. Humar Kahramanli, Novruz Allahverdi, Design of a hybrid system for the diabetes and heart diseases. Expert Syst. Appl. **35**(1-2), 82–89 (2008)
22. I. Abdel-Motaleb, R. Akula, Artificial intelligence algorithm for heart disease diagnosis using phonocardiogram signals, in *2012 IEEE International Conference on Electro/Information Technology* (IEEE, 2012), pp. 1–6
23. S. Ghumbre, C. Patil, A. Ghatol, Heart disease diagnosis using support vector machine, in *International Conference on Computer Science and Information Technology (ICCSIT') Pattaya* (2011)
24. G. Manogaran, R. Varatharajan, M.K. Priyan, Hybrid recommendation system for heart disease diagnosis based on multiple kernel learning with adaptive neuro-fuzzy inference system. Multimedia Tools Appl. **77**(4), 4379–4399 (2018)
25. H. Yan, Y. Jiang, J. Zheng, C. Peng, Q. Li, A multilayer perceptron-based medical decision support system for heart disease diagnosis. Expert Syst. Appl. **30**(2), 272–281 (2006)
26. A. Adeli, M. Neshat, A fuzzy expert system for heart disease diagnosis, in *Proceedings of International Multi Conference of Engineers and Computer Scientists, Hong Kong*, vol. 1 (2010), pp. 28–30
27. J. Nahar, T. Imam, K.S. Tickle, Y.P.P. Chen, Computational intelligence for heart disease diagnosis: A medical knowledge driven approach. Expert Syst. Appl. **40**(1), 96–104 (2013)
28. O.Y. Atkov, S.G. Gorokhova, A.G. Sboev, E.V. Generozov, E.V. Muraseyeva, S.Y. Moroshkina, N.N. Cherniy, Coronary heart disease diagnosis by artificial neural networks including genetic polymorphisms and clinical parameters. J. Cardiol. **59**(2), 190–194 (2012)
29. E.O. Olaniyi, O.K. Oyedotun, K. Adnan, Heart diseases diagnosis using neural networks arbitration. Int. J. Intell. Syst. Appl. **7**(12), 72 (2015)
30. M.G. Feshki, O.S. Shijani, Improving the heart disease diagnosis by evolutionary algorithm of PSO and feed forward neural network, in *2016 Artificial Intelligence and Robotics (IRANOPEN)* (IEEE 2016), pp. 48–53
31. S. Tuli, N. Basumatary, S.S. Gill, M. Kahani, R.C. Arya, G.S. Wander, R. Buyya, Healthfog: an ensemble deep learning based smart healthcare system for automatic diagnosis of heart diseases in integrated IoT and fog computing environments. Future Gener. Comput. Syst. **104**, 187–200 (2020)
32. K.K. Wong, G. Fortino, D. Abbott, Deep learning-based cardiovascular image diagnosis: a promising challenge. Future Gener. Comput. Syst. (2019)
33. R. Alizadehsani, M. Roshanzamir, M. Abdar, A. Beykikhoshk, A. Khosravi, M. Panahiazar, A. Koohestani, N. Sarrafzadegan, A database for using machine learning and data mining techniques for coronary artery disease diagnosis. Sci. Data **6**(1), 1–13 (2019)
34. N. Zhang, G. Yang, Z. Gao, C. Xu, Y. Zhang, R. Shi, J. Keegan, L. Xu, H. Zhang, Z. Fan, D. Firmin, Deep learning for diagnosis of chronic myocardial infarction on nonenhanced cardiac cine MRI. Radiology **291**(3), 606–617 (2019)
35. G.A. Tadesse, T. Zhu, Y. Liu, Y. Zhou, J. Chen, M. Tian, D. Clifton, Cardiovascular disease diagnosis using cross-domain transfer learning, in *2019 41st Annual International Conference of the IEEE Engineering in Medicine and Biology Society (EMBC)* (IEEE, 2019), pp. 4262–4265
36. A.Y. Hannun, P. Rajpurkar, M. Haghpanahi, G.H. Tison, C. Bourn, M.P. Turakhia, A.Y. Ng, Cardiologist-level arrhythmia detection and classification in ambulatory electrocardiograms using a deep neural network. Nat. Med. **25**(1), 65 (2019)
37. A. Junejo, Y. Shen, A.A. Laghari, X. Zhang, H. Luo, Molecular diagnostic and using deep learning techniques for predict functional recovery of patients treated of cardiovascular disease. IEEE Access **7**, 120315–120325 (2019)

38. A. Bhardwaj, A. Kundra, B. Gandhi, S. Kumar, A. Rehalia, M. Gupta, Prediction of heart attack using machine learning. IITM J. Manage. IT **10**(1), 20–24 (2019)
39. B. Ballinger, B., Hsieh, J., Singh, A., Sohoni, N., Wang, J., Tison, G. H., … & Pletcher, M. J. (2018). DeepHeart: semi-supervised sequence learning for cardiovascular risk prediction. In *Thirty-Second AAAI Conference on Artificial Intelligence*
40. A. Kishore, A. Kumar, K. Singh, M. Punia, Y. Hambir, Heart attack prediction using deep learning. Heart **5**(04) (2018)
41. S.B. Patil, Y.S. Kumaraswamy, Extraction of significant patterns from heart disease warehouses for heart attack prediction. IJCSNS **9**(2), 228–235 (2009)
42. R. Chitra, V. Seenivasagam, Heart attack prediction system using fuzzy C means classifier. IOSR J. Comput. Eng. **14**, 23–31 (2013)
43. C. Thirumalai, A. Duba, R. Reddy, Decision making system using machine learning and Pearson for heart attack. In *2017 International Conference of Electronics, Communication and Aerospace Technology (ICECA)*, vol. 2 (IEEE, 2017), pp. 206–210

Chapter 7
A Hybrid Medical Diagnosis Approach with Swarm Intelligence Supported Autoencoder Based Recurrent Neural Network System

Since its first appearance in both academic and scientific world, Artificial Intelligence has taken many steps, which caused to build up different sub-fields focused on different algorithmic solution approaches. It is possible to use Machine Learning based techniques for learning from samples and developing trained intelligent systems [1, 2]. On the other hand, Swarm Intelligence based techniques can be used to solve advanced optimization problems thanks to inspirations from the nature [3, 4]. It is also remarkable that the field of Artificial Intelligence has many relations with alternative computational and engineering oriented fields such as Data Mining, Robotics [5–8]. Among all these complex but flexible solution variations, there has been also a rising interest for building hybrid systems including different Artificial Intelligence techniques-algorithms or traditional solutions to design one, advanced system for solving the target problem. Since the actual task while training a Machine Learning technique is just optimizing its parameters, employing Swarm Intelligence for training phase has been a widely followed hybrid system approach in the associated literature [9–13].

Medical is one of the most remarkable fields in which hybrid Artificial Intelligence based systems are often employed. Because the field of medical is highly open for innovative technological support, Artificial Intelligence based approaches, methods, and techniques have been used widely in the context of hybrid formations, for solving different problems for a long time [14–19]. Today, it is possible to see effective use of Artificial Intelligence based systems for vital problems such as disease diagnosis, medical expert support, information discovery [20–25]. Because sometimes it is difficult to deal with complex and different type of medical data, alternative data processing methods (image/signal processing) [26, 27] and advanced hybrid systems are used as effective and efficient solution ways. It is clear that more advanced use of Artificial Intelligence techniques-algorithms causes better findings for even most complicated problems and data.

This chapter introduces a hybrid system for medical diagnosis. In this sense, a Swarm Intelligence (SI) supported Autoencoder Based Recurrent Neural Network

© The Editor(s) (if applicable) and The Author(s), under exclusive license to Springer Nature Singapore Pte Ltd. 2021
U. Kose et al., *Deep Learning for Medical Decision Support Systems*,
Studies in Computational Intelligence 909,
https://doi.org/10.1007/978-981-15-6325-6_7

(ARNN), which is able to diagnose diseases effectively enough, was designed for ensuring a flexible solution way. Called as SIARNN, the system comes with some codes written with Python programming language and in this way, a fast computational solution approach, which can run pre-defined SI algorithms to feed ARNN with the best resulting data, was obtained accordingly. In this sense, general aim of the SIARNN is to find the optimum, ready-to-use system for achieving good results for the target disease data. The current version the system has a default ARNN model supported by five different well-known and recent SI algorithms: Artificial Bee Colony (ABC), Vortex Optimization Algorithm (VOA), Cuckoo Search (CS), Ant-Lion Optimizer (ALO), and Electro-Search Algorithm (ESA). For understanding more about effectiveness of the SIARNN, it was gone through some evaluation works.

7.1 Related Work

As it was discussed widely so far in the earlier chapters, the associated literature employs many different examples of research employing intelligent systems for medical diagnosis. Here, it is remarkable to indicate that the models of neural networks ensure a great role in the history of artificial intelligence in many problems scopes including especially medical. By giving more consideration to how neural networks have been applied so far, it is possible to provide a wide view for employment of traditional machine learning techniques and then deep learning techniques for different medical diagnosis problems.

In the work by Erkaymaz and his friends [28], general performance of the Small-World Feedforward Neural Networks (SWFNN) was evaluated by considering the diabetes disease. In detail, the work reports that the Newman–Watts small-world model achieved better results than the Watts–Strogatz model. Erkaymaz has also another work with SWFNN to explain some about effect of small-world network topology over conventional ANN structure [29]. The target disease is again diabetes in that work. In another comparative work, the Parkinson disease was diagnosed by using different techniques including also neural networks models [30]. The work reports that the technique of Probabilistic Neural Network (PNN) provided better results than some other classification techniques. In the work [31], Yalcin and her friends examined epilepsy diagnosis by using Electroencephalogram (EEG) time series and running Particle Swarm Optimization (PSO) trained ANN. In the work, ANN-PSO model was compared with alternative models, by considering the epilepsy diagnosis problem. Another example for using EEG data and running intelligent optimization-ANN combination can be seen in the recent work [32] by the author of this study. In detail, the work provides a detailed research over using Ant-Lion Optimizer (ALO) and ANN for studying over EEG time series. Again, the work [33] provides another recent intelligent optimization algorithm: Electro-Search Algorithm (ESA) for training ANFIS that time and working over EEG data. Another work in [34] shows an application of ANN for diagnosing cirrhosis and portal hypertension. But the findings reveal not too much positive effects for use of ANN at the end. As a different disease, the asthma was classified by Badnjević and his friends, by using ANN [35]. According to the work, the model diagnoses the asthma with the success rate of around 97%. As using the feedforward mechanism over a multilayer structure, the research in [36] provides diagnosis for heart diseases, by using ANN. Considering the tuberculosis disease, the work in [37] provides a good, recent review of using Artificial Intelligence and neural networks oriented techniques. In the context of heart diseases, Pandey and Janghel provide a research about use of neural networks model for diagnosing arrhythmia over Electrocardiogram (ECG) data [38]. The work briefly compares Back-Propagation Feedforward Neural Network (BPFNN), Recurrent Neural Network (RNN), and Radial Basis Function Networks (RBF) and shows that RNN has better results according to other models. If we look at to diagnosing diabetes again, it is possible to see use of different Artificial Intelligence techniques. For example, the work [39] provides a research on training Support Vector Machines (SVM) with the Vortex Optimization Algorithm (VOA) for diagnosing diabetes. In another work, Zeng and his friends used SVM and trained it via a variation of PSO: switching-delayed-PSO for diagnosing Alzheimer's disease [40]. For supporting performance of the SVM against diabetes diagnosis, Santhanam, and Padmavathi employed K-Means and Genetic Algorithms (GA) in their work [41]. In the work [42], another example of optimizing SVM can be seen for the diagnosis of coronary artery disease that time. Another effective technique: Random Forest (RF) was used in [43] for diagnosing chronic kidney disease. In the work, RF provided positive results considering its comparison with also alternative classifiers from the literature. A work by Dai and his friends also shows performance of the RF against diagnosing breast cancer [44]. In terms of especially cancer diagnosis, effective use of Deep Learning (DL) is often reported in the literature. The work [45] provides a recent review of image based cancer diagnosis thanks to DL techniques. It is remarkable that the Convolutional Neural Networks (CNN) has been an effective tool for diagnosing cancer over medical image data, as it is effective for dealing with especially image-type data. By benefiting from sonographic images, the work in [46] provides a research of CNN for diagnosing thyroid cancer. The results of the work reveal similar performances by the CNN against even skilled radiologists. On the other hand, the work by Reda and his friends considers the role of DL for early diagnosis of prostate cancer [47]. In the work, applications done over MRI data show a success rate of around 94% with the DL based diagnosis. It is important that especially CNN technique is effective for not only image data but also other types of medical data. In the work by Deperlioglu [48], phonocardiograms were used by CNN for diagnosing heart diseases. Except from CNN, DL has also its different techniques for diagnosing cancer. For example, cancer diagnosis with Deep Belief Networks (DBN) has been reported in many recent works such as [49–52]. From a wider perspective, all DL techniques have very critical role in medical diagnosis as it can be seen even in very recent works of 2019 [53–59]. In the work [60], brain tumor detection and classification was done via ANFIS. A similar research pointing especially detection and segmentation is reported by [61]. Both works have high success rates around 99%. In [62], Yadollahpour and his friends have used the ANFIS for predicting the progression of chronic kidney disease. Here, there seems a remarkable trend for using ANFIS for diagnosis research. For early diagnosis of breast cancer, the work [63] provides a research on using optimized ANFIS focusing on the feature selection issue. As alternative diseases, the works [64] and [65] employ ANFIS model for diagnosing diabetes type 2 and hepatitis, respectively. Both works reveal positive results in terms of using ANFIS for medical diagnosis purposes. In the work [66], Ahmad and his friends use a decision support approach by including ANFIS, k-NN and Information Gain Method. Their system reveals high success rates in terms of diagnosing thyroid diseases. As a recent study, [67] provides the use of VOA for training ANFIS, in order to diagnose thyroid, hepatitis, and chronic kidney diseases. The work reveals positive results in terms of using ANFIS-VOA for medical diagnosis. Another recent work, which was provided by Udoh and his friends, employed ANFIS for diagnosing prostate cancer [68]. The work reports positive results for the ANFIS model. The research in the work [69] introduces the use of ANFIS for the cardio vascular disease. In a very recent work, ANFIS was included in a research for evaluating an introduced prediction method for diagnosing hepatitis disease [70]. In the work [71], Padmavathy and her friends performed a research for breast cancer diagnosis, by employing adaptive clustering, and ANFIS to apply them over mammography images. The results in the work reveal encouraging performance for using ANFIS oriented systems for the target diagnosis problem. The readers are referred to also [72–76] for some other alternative, very recent use of ANFIS within medical diagnosis-oriented applications.

As it can be seen from the mentioned recent works, the literature successfully runs both machine learning and deep learning techniques of artificial intelligence for medical diagnosis. It is also remarkable that the data processing methods such as image processing and signal processing have critical role to make medical data ready for developed solutions. Also, there is a trend of building hybrid systems by simply using the intelligent optimization for training a specific technique performing diagnosis. Considering that, the research in this study is devoted to use of Swarm Intelligence (SI) for training ARNN. It is critical that there is not remarkable use of an ARNN model for solving a disease diagnosis problem. Furthermore, supporting such a model with pre-process through intelligent optimization can be an alternative way to improve medical diagnosis. In this context, the next section explains more about details of the system.

7.2   Swarm Intelligence and Autoencoder Based Recurrent Neural Network for Medical Diagnosis

The solution approach in this chapter is focused on developing an alternative solution environment that can use the advantage of the Autoencoder Based Recurrent Neural Network (ARNN) supported by intelligent optimization. At this point, Swarm Intelligence (SI) techniques-algorithms have been employed for feeding the default ARNN model with better resulting combinations of the data. Since every SI technique may give alternative results for different data sets, an automatic solution mechanism of 'running different SI techniques to have different feature selections for ARNN and choosing the best resulting one' was designed. The system is called as SIARNN as an acronym of SI and ARNN. The following sub-sections give brief information regarding system components (ARNN, SI) and the followed solution approach along with the employed programming approach.

7.2.1   Autoencoder Based Recurrent Neural Network (ARNN)

For understanding more about the model of Autoencoder Based Recurrent Neural Network (ARNN), it is important to explain some about Recurrent Neural Network structure and also Autoencoder mechanism. The model of Recurrent Neural Network (RNN) employs a solution approach, which is for dealing with sequence of input and output data from the internal states. Thus, a system structure, which is acting like a memory, is designed [77, 78]. Moving from that, it can be said that the RNN model is used effectively when it is important to understand something from sequence of the data. Figure 7.1 shows the model structure for the RNN [78].

Data processing through a RNN is as follows [78]:

- At the time of t, o_t corresponds to the output while x_t is for the input. The memory of the neural network is defined with s_t, which is the hidden state at the time: t.
- By using a function such as *ReLU* or *tanh*, s_t is get via $f(Ux_t + Ws_{t-1})$, where the current input and the previous hidden state are enrolled (As default, s_{-1} is set as all zeroes).

In the study here, an RNN model was combined with the Autoencoder. Autoencoder is a type of neural network, which can be used for reducing high dimensionality of the target data. Thanks to learning low level representation of the input(s),

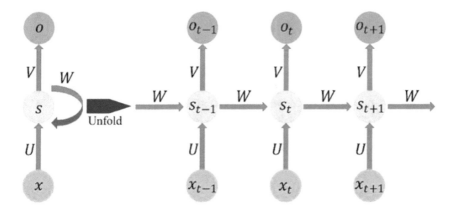

Fig. 7.1   A typical RNN model structure [78]

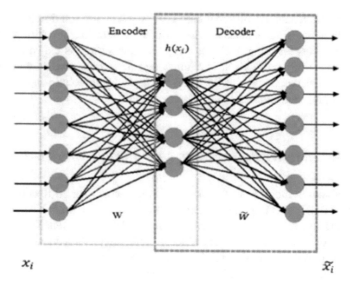

Fig. 7.2   A typical autoencoder model structure [80]

Autoencoder is useful for especially solving complex problems. A typical Autoencoder model includes three layers of input, hidden, and output, where same number of neurons for input(s) and output(s) is used. In the system structure, input and hidden layers run an encoding scheme whereas hidden and output layers are for decoding, leading to low dimension of target data [79, 80]. Figure 7.2 shows a typical representation of an Autoencoder model [80].

7.2.2   Swarm Intelligence and Intelligent Optimization in the SIARNN

Because traditional optimization methods are not enough to solve more complicated optimization problems, intelligent optimization methods by Artificial Intelligence have been used effectively for a while. Since the real life is actually a mixture of optimization problems, intelligent optimization is widely used in all fields with different optimization-oriented perspectives such as continuous optimization and combinatorial optimization. Currently, there are many different intelligent optimization-based algorithms-techniques, which are inspired from different components of the nature [81]. So, it is possible to classify these algorithms-techniques under different titles. But the most comprehensive one is Swarm Intelligence (SI). As a sub-field of Artificial Intelligence, the concept of SI refers to collective, interactive problem-solving behaviors of a group of (mostly) living organisms such as animals, insects or even humans [82, 83]. In terms of algorithmic design, Artificial Intelligence ensures mathematical and logical steps to simulate the related behaviors under iterative optimization processes. In this way, modeled real life optimization problems are solved by some particles, whose parameters can change relative to state of each other in the swarm [81, 84].

The infrastructure of the SIARNN is based on training an ARNN model via SI techniques. But because there is always a competitive state among different SI techniques to have better solutions for target problems, SIARNN has been structured to include running different SI techniques over same ARNN model to find the best solution for a specific medical diagnosis data. In this context, SIARNN considers the following rules for diagnosis process:

- Read the target disease diagnosis data to determine the complexity of the target disease,
- List and determine the past best-performing SI techniques for the target disease,
- Based on default or user-defined parameters, start to perform feature extraction with each SI technique and feed the ARNN,
- Evaluate performance of each hybrid ARNN-SI combination for diagnosing the target disease.

Based on the mentioned rules, default running algorithm of the SIARNN is presented in Fig. 7.3.

The feature selection by each SI technique is accomplished via particles by evaluating results of different features over evaluation metric(s) (i.e. Equation 2: *Accuracy*

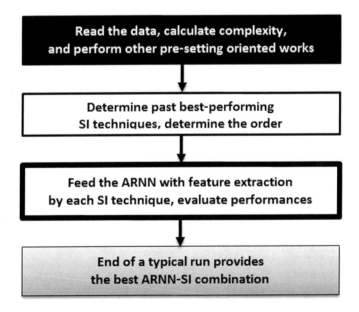

Fig. 7.3 Running algorithm of the SIARNN

in this study) regarding the diagnosis by the ARNN (the diagnosis in this study was a typical classification approach).

The SIARNN system in the research of this study included five different SI techniques. Essentials of these techniques have been explained briefly as follows:

7.2.2.1   Artificial Bee Colony

Artificial Bee Colony (ABC) is a popular intelligent optimization technique, which was introduced by Karaboga and Basturk [85]. ABC briefly inspires from honey bees and provides a role based approach for dealing with advanced optimization problems. In detail, ABC employs optimization processes as a simple, mathematical simulation of food search behavior shown by bees. Essential features of the ABC can be expressed briefly as follows [85–87]:

- The algorithm flow is associated with interaction among particles (bees) and food-nectar sources corresponding to values found within the solution space.
- There are three roles for the particles-bees; a bee can be employed bee, onlooker bee, or scout bee. As general, all of the bees search for optimum value(s) by interacting each other.
- After employed bees find some values-nectar, they perform dance moves to attract onlooker bees and if it is appropriate, some of onlooker bees become employed bees by taking place in employed bees' places.
- Out of interactions among employed and onlooker bees, scout bees just randomly search for better value(s). Along the algorithm process, employed bees, who cannot be improved more, are transformed into scout bees.

Regarding the ABC, more information can be obtained from sources: [85, 87, 88].

7.2.2.2   Vortex Optimization Algorithm

As introduced by Kose and Arslan [89, 90], Vortex Optimization Algorithm (VOA) is based on the dynamics of vortices in the nature. As not being based on a specific type of living organisms, VOA considers the particles as in the role of 'normal flows' or 'vortices'. According to the state of a particle, evolution-oriented elimination mechanism of the technique tries to get good particles effective enough to find desired optimum solution(s). Some of remarkable features of the VOA can be mentioned as follows [89, 90]:

- Through the iterative process, role of a particle may be change to the normal flow or vortex, according to its performance.
- Vortices have better values according to normal flows. So, normal flows-particles tend to move towards vortices.
- The whole particle population is refreshed partially by eliminating worst particles and locating new particles in the solution space.

- The VOA also employs an in-system optimization approach for dealing with difficult, advanced optimization problems.

For more details regarding the VOA, readers can examine the sources: [89–91].

7.2.2.3   Cuckoo Search

Cuckoo Search (CS) is another intelligent optimization technique as based on brood parasitism behavior shown by some cuckoo species. CS was introduced by Yang and Deb [92] and it is mostly focused on cuckoo breeding as associated with parasitism. Along the optimization process, particles (cuckoos) try to continue their breeding by going through variable values, which are nests with eggs. In this sense, some features of the CS are as follows [92, 93]:

- Each cuckoo can have one egg and that egg can be placed to a random nest during the searching within solution space. At this point, nests are found values by cuckoos, as thought to be optimum solution(s).
- Thanks to some mathematical and logical steps, cuckoos try to find better nests and eliminate foreign eggs. Better values-nests are taken to next generations during the algorithmic process.
- It is remarkable that the searching mechanism in the CS is done via Levy Flights, which is a type of random searching mechanism, inspired by movements of many living organisms in the life [94].

More details regarding the algorithmic structure and solution mechanism of the CS can be found at [92, 95, 96].

7.2.2.4   Ant-Lion Optimizer

Ant-Lion Optimizer (ALO) is a very recent technique-algorithm for intelligent optimization. As developed by Mirjalili [97], ALO employs solution mechanism by simulating hunting behaviors of ant-lions during their larvae stage. Briefly, ant-lions build traps under the ground, in order to hunt ants. That behavior is the cause for calling these insects as ant-lion. The ALO includes algorithmic steps for ensuring interaction among ants and ant-lions, which are particles to search and keep potential optimum values. Considering the algorithm, some important points are as follows [98, 99]:

- Both ant-lions and ants are responsible for searching values within the solution space.
- During searching, a random walk approach is used for changing positions-values.
- Ant-lions' behavior of trapping ants is just adapting an ant-lion's position (values for calculating fitness) to the target ant, which seems having good value(s).

More details for that recent algorithm can be found at the sources: [97–99].

7.2.2.5   Electro-Search Algorithm

As introduced by Tabari and Ahmad [100], Electro-Search Algorithm (ESA) is the most recent technique employed in the research in this study. ESA briefly considers movements of electrons with orbits around an atom nucleus and provides an algorithmic way for optimization problems. The solution process is a mixture of locating particles (atoms), transitions among orbits, and updating nucleus locations. Some remarkable features of the ESA are as follows [100]:

- ESA uses mathematical mechanism in some known principles like Bohr Model or Rydberg Formula, and provides a well-structured solution process.
- Atoms are potential solutions in which orbits of electrons and nucleus positions are components-value(s) determined during the optimization process.
- ESA employs an in-system optimization approach called as Orbital-Tuner for ensuring that the initial parameter values do not affect the performance directly (like other SI techniques-algorithms).

Readers are referred to [100] for more details about ESA.

Considering the explained SI techniques-algorithms, the SIARNN has been developed by using Python programming language. Here, a modular approach was followed for efficient use. The next sub-section expresses some about general design of the SIARNN in this manner.

7.3   Design of the SIARNN

SIARNN has been coded by using Python programming language, which was thought as a fast and comprehensive enough environment to run a system consisting of different Artificial Intelligence techniques running collaboratively. As like many similar applications done via Python, some well-known libraries were also included while designing the whole SIARNN mechanism. For further versions of the system and performance-adjusting code additions, a modular approach, which follows the use of separate code files-modules, was build. Some of remarkable design notes for the SIARNN are as follows:

- *Numpy*, and *SciPy* are two well-known Python libraries used in the SIARNN, for especially mathematical-scientific calculations during solution processes.
- SIARNN employs the *Root.py* file as the central control mechanism of the system. All other modules including Artificial Intelligence side are connected to that file.
- *DataProblemSet.py* is used for evaluating the target data set, calculating the complexity, and setting the initial problem variables or SI technique components before running the optimization. The following complexity calculation is used for each target disease data set:

$$Complexity = OutputClass * \left[(2 * Numeric) + (\sum_{i=1}^{N} Nominal_i) \right] \quad (1)$$

In Eq. (1), *OutputClass* stands for total number of classes under the output attribute, *Numeric* stands for total number of input attributes having numeric-real numbers, and *Nominal* is for total number of classes for each input attributes having nominal values. As it can be understood, the diversity in terms of different classes or number of numerical attributes causes more complexity. The calculated value is later used by the system to improve efficiency of the system in new applications. If a disease data, which was evaluated before, is used again for diagnosis, the SI technique having the highest success point is used directly (if the user only wants the SIARNN to perform diagnosis for target input data). Otherwise, the order of the SI techniques to run with the ARNN is determined according to similarities between past complexity values solved by each SI technique and the current complexity value. Equivalence in similarities causes random order or determining the order according to success points and/or rankings.

- *Performance.py* is used for detecting the best performing ARNN-SI combination and storing the data for past diagnosis performances. Stored data includes ranking of each SI technique for target disease data, general success point of each SI technique (1st takes 4 point, 2nd takes 2 point, and 3rd takes 1 point while the other ones takes 0 point), and complexity for the used disease data set.
- ARNN and SI techniques are in separate file forms. As long as the parameters of *Root.py* and *ProblemSet.py* are met, separate SI techniques can be coded as separate .py files to be included within the SIARNN infrastructure.

Figure 7.4 presents a general scheme of the SIARNN code design and relation among the SIARNN modules.

Thanks to current Python code design, SIARNN can be run by just giving appropriate parameters over console. For unexperienced users of SIARNN, it is possible to run the system by feeding with some specific parameters (such as particle numbers, iteration number) and the target data but the system allows advanced users to determine any specific parameters such as parameters for each different SI techniques-algorithms or ARNN model.

7.4 Applications and Evaluation

It is important to have idea about the performance of SIARNN in the context of medical diagnosis. In order to achieve that, the SIARNN has been applied to several medical disease data sets and the best-performing values of the SIARNN were evaluated accordingly. Additionally, those best-performing values were compared with the performances by some alternative techniques. The next sub-sections provide information about all these stages.

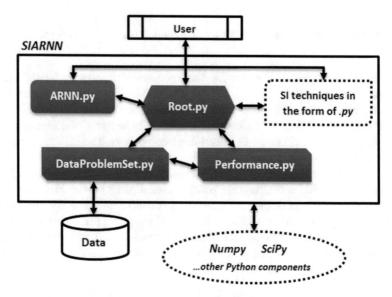

Fig. 7.4 Design of the SIARNN in terms of code infrastructure

7.4.1 Medical Diagnosis Applications with SIARNN

Medical diagnosis performance of the SIARNN has been evaluated by considering four different disease data sets from UCI Machine Learning Repository [101]. As the first data set, Pima Indians Diabetes includes 8 attributes with 614 training, and 154 test data. As the second data set, the Thyroid includes 21 attributes, and provides 2800 training, and 972 test data. The third data set, Hepatitis employs 19 attributes within 100 training, and 55 test data. Finally, the Chronic Kidney Disease data set is based on 25 attributes within 295 training, and 105 test data. All data sets classify the corresponding values for their input attributes as 0: healthy person, or 1: person with disease at the output attribute.

For the diagnosis applications, all SI techniques employed 120 particles and their parameters were set to default values reported in the literature. After feature extraction phases in each disease data set, performance of the SIARNN with different SI technique was evaluated with the test data, by considering the simple accuracy rate calculation in Eq. (2). In the related equation, *TC* stands for true classification of the target data (whether it is 0 or 1 at the output), and *FC* for false classification:

$$Accuracy = 100 * \frac{TC}{TC + FC} \tag{2}$$

Based on each of five SI techniques, diagnosis performance of SIARNN systems is provided in Table 7.1. As it is known, SIARNN has determined the best-performing ARNN-SI combination at the end of running different combinations. So, Table 7.1

Table 7.1 SIARNN performances in each medical diagnosis application

Application/disease	Accuracy rate/rank[a] for;				
	ARNN-ABC	ARNN-VOA	ARNN-CS	ARNN-ALO	ARNN-ESA
Pima Indian diabetes	98.05/2	97.40/3	98.70/1	97.40/3	97.40/3
Thyroid	97.42/2	97.02/4	97.33/3	97.63/1	97.02/4
Hepatitis	92.73/4	94.55/3	96.36/2	98.18/1	92.73/4
Chronic kidney	92.38/3	90.48/5	94.29/1	93.33/2	91.43/4

[a]Best values in bold

shows accuracy rates and ranking for all five ARNN-SI combination of the SIARNN while the values for the chosen-best (ranked as 1) combination in each disease data set (diagnosis) are shown in bold style.

Moving from Table 7.1, it is possible to express that there are good performances by different ARNN-SI combinations for diagnosing four different diseases. However, ARNN models with ALO, and CS outperform other ones generally.

7.4.2 Comparative Evaluation

For evaluating the SIARNN further, it was compared with some additional Artificial Intelligence techniques. At this point, the best-performing findings by ARNN-ALO and ARNN-CS (Table 7.1) were compared with the performances by four additional techniques. In this context, traditional Multi-Layer Perceptron Artificial Neural Networks model trained via Back-Propagation Algorithm (ANN-BPA) [102, 103], default ANFIS model trained by hybrid Gradient Descent and Least Squares Estimator (ANFIS-GDLSE) [104, 105], Support Vector Machines (SVM) [106, 107], and K-Nearest Neighbor algorithm (K-NN) [108, 109] were included for the comparison. Findings in terms of diagnosis accuracy rate of each technique are presented in Table 7.2 (best values are shown in bold style).

As it can be seen from Table 7.2, best-performing SIARNN findings are generally better than alternative techniques from the literature. By considering both Tables 7.1,

Table 7.2 Comparative evaluation with SIARNN, ANN-BPA, ANFIS-GDLSE, SVM, and K-NN

Application/disease	Accuracy rate[a] for;				
	SIARNN	ANN-BPA	ANFIS-GDLSE	SVM	K-NN
Pima Indian diabetes	98.70 (ARNN-CS)	96.10	98.05	98.70	94.16
Thyroid	97.63 (ARNN-ALO)	97.33	97.42	97.74	97.02
Hepatitis	98.18 (ARNN-ALO)	92.73	94.55	96.36	90.91
Chronic kidney	94.29 (ARNN-CS)	90.48	91.43	93.33	87.62

[a]Best values in bold

and 7.2, it is possible to express that the formed SIARNN system is able to perform effective medical diagnosis for different disease data sets. Furthermore, it is easy to work with SIARNN since it can determine the best-performing ARNN-SI combination for the target data set. That advantage is important for especially users, who do not know what type of Artificial Intelligence oriented system is working on the background but wait for good enough diagnosis performance by the computer assistance.

7.5 Results and Future Work

In this chapter, a Swarm Intelligence (SI) supported Autoencoder Based Recurrent Neural Network (ARNN) has been introduced for medical diagnosis processes. In detail, the system includes some pre-defined SI algorithms for performing feature extraction sessions to feed ARNN against the target data set. It automatically detects the best performing ARNN and SI combination for better results at the end. The system was coded with the Python programming language in a modular way and it was supported with five different SI algorithms: Artificial Bee Colony (ABC), Vortex Optimization Algorithm (VOA), Cuckoo Search (CS), Ant-Lion Optimizer (ALO), and Electro-Search Algorithm (ESA). Called as briefly Swarm Intelligence supported Autoencoder Based Recurrent Neural Network (SIARNN), it is a typical medical diagnosis environment, which can be improved in future versions.

In order to understand more about success of the SIARNN, it was evaluated by using four different medical disease data sets. According to the findings, SIARNN can diagnose target diseases successfully thanks to flexible infrastructure allowing detection of the best ARNN and SI algorithm combination. It was seen that the SIARNN with especially ALO and CS can achieve better diagnosis rather than other SI techniques-algorithms. Additionally, comparison done with SIARNN and some other Artificial Intelligence techniques showed that the SIARNN can be an effective tool for intelligent medical diagnosis.

Especially positive results are important signs for thinking about future works. In this context, the SIARNN can be supported with additional SI algorithms and new modules (in terms of programming) for new features and functions (i.e. in-system parameter optimization, flexible neural networks structure). Also, the system can be evaluated with additional data sets in order to understand more about the success over different diseases. On the other hand, there can be more evaluation tasks for different cases such as general process time and performance against different medical data types, system flexibility against different sources...etc. Finally, there can be also future efforts to develop similar medical diagnosis systems by including alternative Deep Learning (DL) oriented neural networks.

7.6 Summary

It is important that the field of artificial intelligence has always been enrolled in strong relations with different research areas related to especially data processing approaches. Because machine/deep learning processes are actually optimization problems to be solved, algorithms—techniques for optimization have been also employed for improving capabilities of the known techniques. In accordance to that, swarm intelligence has been a successful tool for designing hybrid systems, in addition to alternative hybrid systems formation approaches done by using computational techniques out of the field of artificial intelligence.

This chapter provided a typical use of a Swarm Intelligence (SI) within a deep learning solution for medical diagnosis leading to decision support. In this sense, an Autoencoder Based Recurrent Neural Network (ARNN) has been introduced for medical diagnosis processes, as trained by the SI. Called as briefly Swarm Intelligence supported Autoencoder Based Recurrent Neural Network (SIARNN), the developed system includes some pre-defined SI algorithms for ensuring feature extraction sessions to feed ARNN against the target data set. It automatically detects the best performing ARNN and SI combination for better results at the end. It is critical that the SIARNN was used for different diagnosis data sets and it provided successful enough results for achieving a multi-disease/multi-diagnosis solution at the end. The system was coded with the Python programming language in a modular way and its current version includes five different SI algorithms: Artificial Bee Colony (ABC), Vortex Optimization Algorithm (VOA), Cuckoo Search (CS), Ant-Lion Optimizer (ALO), and Electro-Search Algorithm (ESA). Of course, it is open for future improvements for better diagnosis rates and forming a bigger diagnosis environment.

As the chapters so far have shown diagnosis support of deep learning solutions for the diseases with generally known symptoms and signs to be analyzed with physical ways. On the other hand, one important use of medical decision support systems has been in the context of psychological approaches since people also have mental and psychological problems because of different factors. As that is a very specific, different and complex way of medical diagnosis, the role of deep learning should also be explained accordingly. In this context, the Chap. 8 in the next pages provides a psychological personal support system based on a deep learning approach.

7.7 Further Learning

In order to have more information about intelligent optimization, and the associated subjects such as swarm intelligence, evolutionary computing, heuristics and metaheuristics, the readers can read [110–120].

As very recent alternative swarm intelligence techniques—algorithms, the readers can take a look at to [121–125].

For very recent applications of hybrid systems with use of machine/deep learning techniques, the readers are referred to [126–134].

References

1. E. Alpaydin, *Introduction to Machine Learning* (MIT Press, Cambridge, MA, 2009)
2. P. Harrington, *Machine Learning in Action* (Manning Publications Co., New York, US, 2012)
3. E. Bonabeau, D.D.R.D.F. Marco, M. Dorigo, G. Theraulaz, *Swarm Intelligence: From Natural to Artificial Systems (No. 1)* (Oxford University Press, Oxford, 1999)
4. X.S. Yang, Z. Cui, R. Xiao, A.H. Gandomi, M. Karamanoglu (eds.), *Swarm Intelligence and Bio-inspired Computation: Theory and Applications* (Newnes, London, 2013)
5. G. Lakemeyer, B. Nebel (eds.), *Exploring Artificial Intelligence in the New Millennium* (Morgan Kaufmann, Los Altos, CA, 2003)
6. B. Thuraisingham, Data Mining: Technologies, Techniques, Tools, and Trends. (CRC Press, London, 2014)
7. M. Brady, L.A. Gerhardt, H.F. Davidson (eds.), *Robotics and Artificial Intelligence*, vol. 11 (Springer, New York, 2012)
8. A. Ghosal, *Robotics: Fundamental Concepts and Analysis* (Oxford University Press, Oxford, 2006)
9. A. Abraham, E. Corchado, J.M. Corchado, Hybrid learning machines. Neurocomputing **72**(13–15), 2729–2730 (2009)
10. S. Wermter, *Hybrid Neural Systems (No. 1778)* (Springer, New York, 2000)
11. L.R. Medsker, *Hybrid Intelligent Systems* (Springer, New York, 2012)
12. C. Grosan, A. Abraham, Hybrid evolutionary algorithms: methodologies, architectures, and reviews, *Hybrid Evolutionary Algorithms* (Springer, Berlin, Heidelberg, 2007), pp. 1–17
13. S. Sahin, M.R. Tolun, R. Hassanpour, Hybrid expert systems: A survey of current approaches and applications. Expert Syst. Appl. **39**(4), 4609–4617 (2012)
14. F. Jiang, Y. Jiang, H. Zhi, Y. Dong, H. Li, S. Ma, …, Y. Wang, Artificial intelligence in healthcare: past, present and future. Stroke Vasc. Neurol. **2**(4), 230–243 (2017)
15. P.L. Miller (ed.), *Selected Topics in Medical Artificial Intelligence* (Springer, New York, 2012)
16. D.D. Luxton (ed.), *Artificial Intelligence in Behavioral and Mental Health Care* (Elsevier, Amsterdam, 2015)
17. P. Hamet, J. Tremblay, Artificial intelligence in medicine. Metabolism **69**, S36–S40 (2017)
18. P.J. Lisboa, A.F. Taktak, The use of artificial neural networks in decision support in cancer: A systematic review. Neural Networks **19**(4), 408–415 (2006)
19. M. Hengstler, E. Enkel, S. Duelli, Applied artificial intelligence and trust—the case of autonomous vehicles and medical assistance devices. Technol. Forecast. Soc. Chang. **105**, 105–120 (2016)
20. F. Amato, A. López, E.M. Peña-Méndez, P. Vaňhara, A. Hampl, J. Havel, Artificial neural networks in medical diagnosis. J. Appl. Biomed. **11**(2), 47–58 (2013)
21. Q.K. Al-Shayea, Artificial neural networks in medical diagnosis. Int. J. Comput. Sci. Issues **8**(2), 150–154 (2011)
22. E.H. Shortliffe, M.J. Sepúlveda, Clinical decision support in the era of artificial intelligence. JAMA **320**(21), 2199–2200 (2018)
23. C.C. Bennett, T.W. Doub, Expert systems in mental health care: AI applications in decision-making and consultation, *Artificial Intelligence in Behavioral and Mental Health Care* (Academic Press, London, 2016), pp. 27–51
24. C. Yao, Y. Qu, B. Jin, L. Guo, C. Li, W. Cui, L. Feng, A convolutional neural network model for online medical guidance. IEEE Access **4**, 4094–4103 (2016)
25. Y. Jing, Y. Bian, Z. Hu, L. Wang, X.Q.S. Xie, Deep learning for drug design: an artificial intelligence paradigm for drug discovery in the big data era. AAPS J **20**(3), 58 (2018)

26. A.C. Bovik, Handbook of Image and Video Processing. (Elsevier Academic Press, 2010)
27. T.K. Moon, W.C. Stirling, *Mathematical Methods and Algorithms for Signal Processing (Vol. 1)* (Prentice Hall, Upper Saddle River, NJ, 2000)
28. O. Erkaymaz, M. Ozer, M. Perc, Performance of small-world feedforward neural networks for the diagnosis of diabetes. Appl. Math. Comput. **311**, 22–28 (2017)
29. O. Erkaymaz, M. Ozer, Impact of small-world network topology on the conventional artificial neural network for the diagnosis of diabetes. Chaos, Solitons Fractals **83**, 178–185 (2016)
30. O. Er, O. Cetin, M.S. Bascil, F. Temurtas, A Comparative study on Parkinson's disease diagnosis using neural networks and artificial immune system. J. Med. Imaging Health Inf. **6**(1), 264–268 (2016)
31. N. Yalcin, G. Tezel, C. Karakuzu, Epilepsy diagnosis using artificial neural network learned by PSO. Turk. J. Electr. Eng. Comput. Sci. **23**(2), 421–432 (2015)
32. U. Kose, An Ant-Lion optimizer-trained artificial neural network system for chaotic electroencephalogram (EEG) Prediction. Appl. Sci. **8**(9), 1613 (2018)
33. J.A.M. Saucedo, J.D. Hemanth, U. Kose, Prediction of electroencephalogram time series with electro-search optimization algorithm trained adaptive neuro-fuzzy inference system. IEEE Access **7**, 15832–15844 (2019)
34. B. Procopet, V.M. Cristea, M.A. Robic, M. Grigorescu, P.S. Agachi, S. Metivier, … J.P. Vinel, "Serum tests, liver stiffness and artificial neural networks for diagnosing cirrhosis and portal hypertension. Dig. Liver Dis. **47**(5), 411–416 (2015)
35. A. Badnjević, L. Gurbeta, M. Cifrek, D. Marjanovic, Classification of asthma using artificial neural network, in *2016 39th International Convention on Information and Communication Technology, Electronics and Microelectronics (MIPRO)*. (IEEE, 2016), pp. 387–390
36. E.O. Olaniyi, O.K. Oyedotun, K. Adnan, Heart diseases diagnosis using neural networks arbitration. Int. J. Intell. Syst. Appl. **7**(12), 72 (2015)
37. P. Dande, P. Samant, Acquaintance to artificial Neural Networks and use of artificial intelligence as a diagnostic tool for tuberculosis: a review. Tuberculosis **108**, 1–9 (2018)
38. S.K. Pandey, R.R. Janghel, ECG arrhythmia classification using artificial neural networks, in *Proceedings of 2nd International Conference on Communication, Computing and Networking*. (Springer, Singapore, 2019), pp. 645–652
39. S.F. Cankaya, I.A. Cankaya, T. Yigit, A. Koyun, Diabetes diagnosis system based on support vector machines trained by vortex optimization algorithm, in *Nature-Inspired Intelligent Techniques for Solving Biomedical Engineering Problems*. (IGI Global, 2018), pp. 203–218
40. N. Zeng, H. Qiu, Z. Wang, W. Liu, H. Zhang, Y. Li, A new switching-delayed-PSO-based optimized SVM algorithm for diagnosis of Alzheimer's disease. Neurocomputing **320**, 195–202 (2018)
41. T. Santhanam, M.S. Padmavathi, Application of K-means and genetic algorithms for dimension reduction by integrating SVM for diabetes diagnosis. Proc. Comput. Sci. **47**, 76–83 (2015)
42. A.D. Dolatabadi, S.E.Z. Khadem, B.M. Asl, Automated diagnosis of coronary artery disease (CAD) patients using optimized SVM. Comput. Methods Programs Biomed. **138**, 117–126 (2017)
43. A. Subasi, E. Alickovic, J. Kevric, Diagnosis of chronic kidney disease by using random forest, in *CMBEBIH 2017*. (Springer, Singapore, 2017), pp. 589–594
44. B. Dai, R.C. Chen, S.Z. Zhu, W.W. Zhang, Using random forest algorithm for breast cancer diagnosis, in *2018 International Symposium on Computer, Consumer and Control (IS3C)*. (IEEE, 2018), pp. 449–452
45. Z. Hu, J. Tang, Z. Wang, K. Zhang, L. Zhang, Q. Sun, Deep learning for image-based cancer detection and diagnosis—a survey. Pattern Recogn. **83**, 134–149 (2018)
46. X. Li, S. Zhang, Q. Zhang, X. Wei, Y. Pan, J. Zhao, …, F. Yang, Diagnosis of thyroid cancer using deep convolutional neural network models applied to sonographic images: a retrospective, multicohort, diagnostic study. Lancet Oncol. **20**(2), 193–201 (2019)
47. I. Reda, A. Khalil, M. Elmogy, A. Abou El-Fetouh, A. Shalaby, M. Abou El-Ghar, …, A. El-Baz, Deep learning role in early diagnosis of prostate cancer. Technol. Cancer Res. Treat. **17**, 1533034618775530 (2018)

48. O. Deperlioglu, Classification of phonocardiograms with convolutional neural networks. BRAIN. Broad Res. Artif. Intell. Neurosci. **9**(2), 22–33 (2018)
49. J.R. Burt, N. Torosdagli, N. Khosravan, H. RaviPrakash, A. Mortazi, F. Tissavirasingham, …, U. Bagci, Deep learning beyond cats and dogs: recent advances in diagnosing breast cancer with deep neural networks. British J. Radiol. **91**(1089), 20170545 (2018)
50. S. Azizi, F. Imani, B. Zhuang, A. Tahmasebi, J.T. Kwak, S. Xu, …, B. Wood, Ultrasound-based detection of prostate cancer using automatic feature selection with deep belief networks. in *International Conference on Medical Image Computing and Computer-Assisted Intervention.* (Springer, Cham, 2015), pp. 70–77
51. A.M. Abdel-Zaher, A.M. Eldeib, Breast cancer classification using deep belief networks. Expert Syst. Appl. **46**, 139–144 (2016)
52. M.A. Al-antari, M.A. Al-masni, S.U. Park, J. Park, M.K. Metwally, Y.M. Kadah, …, T.S. Kim, An automatic computer-aided diagnosis system for breast cancer in digital mammograms via deep belief network. J. Med. Biol. Eng. **38**(3), 443–456 (2018)
53. S. Khan, N. Islam, Z. Jan, I.U. Din, J.J.C. Rodrigues, A novel deep learning based framework for the detection and classification of breast cancer using transfer learning. Pattern Recogn. Lett. **125**, 1–6 (2019)
54. C.J. Wang, C.A. Hamm, B.S. Letzen, J.S. Duncan, A probabilistic approach for interpretable deep learning in liver cancer diagnosis, in *Medical Imaging 2019: Computer-Aided Diagnosis* (Vol. 10950). (International Society for Optics and Photonics, 2019), p. 109500U
55. A. Yala, C. Lehman, T. Schuster, T. Portnoi, R. Barzilay, A deep learning mammography-based model for improved breast cancer risk prediction. Radiology, 182716 (2019)
56. E.J. Ha, J.H. Baek, D.G. Na, Deep convolutional neural network models for the diagnosis of thyroid cancer. Lancet Oncol. **20**(3), e130 (2019)
57. A. Cheng, Y. Kim, E. M. Anas, A. Rahmim, E.M. Boctor, R. Seifabadi, B.J. Wood, Deep learning image reconstruction method for limited-angle ultrasound tomography in prostate cancer, in *Medical Imaging 2019: Ultrasonic Imaging and Tomography*, vol. 10955. (International Society for Optics and Photonics, 2019), p. 1095516
58. A. Kharrat, M. Néji, Classification of brain tumors using personalized deep belief networks on MRImages: PDBN-MRI, in *11th International Conference on Machine Vision (ICMV 2018)*, vol. 11041. (International Society for Optics and Photonics, 2019), p. 110412 M
59. N.A. Ali, A.R. Syafeeza, L.J. Geok, Y.C. Wong, N.A. Hamid, A.S. Jaafar, *Design of automated computer-aided classification of brain tumor using deep learning, in Intelligent and Interactive Computing* (Springer, Singapore, 2019), pp. 285–291
60. P. Thirumurugan, P. Shanthakumar, Brain tumor detection and diagnosis using ANFIS classifier. Int. J. Imaging Syst. Technol. **26**(2), 157–162 (2016)
61. S. Kumarganesh, M. Suganthi, An enhanced medical diagnosis sustainable system for brain tumor detection and segmentation using ANFIS classifier. Curr. Med. Imaging Rev. **14**(2), 271–279 (2018)
62. A. Yadollahpour, J. Nourozi, S.A. Mirbagheri, E. Simancas-Acevedo, F.R. Trejo-Macotela, Designing and implementing an ANFIS based medical decision support system to predict chronic kidney disease progression. Frontiers Physiol. **9** (2018)
63. A. Addeh, H. Demirel, P. Zarbakhsh, Early detection of breast cancer using optimized anfis and features selection, in *2017 9th International Conference on Computational Intelligence and Communication Networks (CICN)*. (IEEE, 2017), pp. 39–42
64. M. Kirisci, H. Yılmaz, M.U. Saka, An ANFIS perspective for the diagnosis of type II diabetes. *Annals of Fuzzy Mathematics and Informatics*. (In Press, afmi.or.kr, 2019)
65. W. Ahmad, A. Ahmad, A. Iqbal, M. Hamayun, A. Hussain, G. Rehman, …, L. Huang, Intelligent hepatitis diagnosis using adaptive neuro-fuzzy inference system and information gain method. Soft Comput. 1–8 (2018)
66. W. Ahmad, L. Huang, A. Ahmad, F. Shah, A. Iqbal, Thyroid diseases forecasting using a hybrid decision support system based on ANFIS, k-NN and information gain method. J. Appl. Environ. Biol. Sci. **7**, 78–85 (2017)

67. T. Yigit, S. Celik, Intelligent disease diagnosis with vortex optimization algorithm based ANFIS. J. Multi. Dev. **3**(1), 1–20 (2019)
68. S.S. Udoh, U.A. Umoh, M.E. Umoh, M.E. Udo, Diagnosis of prostate cancer using soft computing paradigms. Global J. Comput. Sci. Technol. **19**(2), 19–26 (2019)
69. L. Sarangi, M.N. Mohanty, S. Patnaik, Design of ANFIS based e-health care system for cardio vascular disease detection, in *International Conference on Intelligent and Interactive Systems and Applications*. (Springer, Cham, 2016), pp. 445–453
70. M. Nilashi, H. Ahmadi, L. Shahmoradi, O. Ibrahim, E. Akbari, A predictive method for hepatitis disease diagnosis using ensembles of neuro-fuzzy technique. J. Inf. Pub. Health **12**(1), 13–20 (2019)
71. T.V. Padmavathy, M.N. Vimalkumar, D.S. Bhargava, Adaptive clustering based breast cancer detection with ANFIS classifier using mammographic images". Clust. Comput. 1–10 (2018)
72. W. Rajab, S. Rajab, V. Sharma, Kernel FCM-based ANFIS approach to heart disease prediction, in *Emerging Trends in Expert Applications and Security*. (Springer, Singapore, 2019), pp. 643–650
73. E.K. Roy, S.K. Aditya, Prediction of acute myeloid leukemia subtypes based on artificial neural network and adaptive neuro-fuzzy inference system approaches, in *Innovations in Electronics and Communication Engineering*. (Springer, Singapore, 2019), pp. 427–439
74. M. Imran, S.A. Alsuhaibani, A neuro-fuzzy inference model for diabetic retinopathy classification, in *Intelligent Data Analysis for Biomedical Applications*. (Academic Press, London, 2019), pp. 147–172
75. S. Zainuddin, F. Nhita, U.N. Wisesty, Classification of gene expressions of lung cancer and colon tumor using adaptive-network-based fuzzy inference system (ANFIS) with ant colony optimization (ACO) as the feature selection, in *Journal of Physics: Conference Series*, vol. 1192, no. 1. (IOP Publishing, 2019), p. 012019
76. M.N. Fata, R. Arifudin, B. Prasetiyo, Optimization neuro fuzzy using genetic algorithm for diagnose typhoid fever. Sci. J. Inf. **6**(1), 1–11 (2019)
77. B.S. Babu, A. Suneetha, G.C. Babu, Y.J.N. Kumar, G. Karuna, Medical disease prediction using grey wolf optimization and auto encoder based recurrent neural network. Period. Eng. and Nat. Sci. **6**(1), 229–240 (2018)
78. W. Bao, J. Yue, Y. Rao, A deep learning framework for financial time series using stacked auto encoders and long-short term memory. PLoS ONE **12**(7), e0180944 (2017)
79. P. Baldi, Autoencoders, unsupervised learning, and deep architectures, in *Proceedings of ICML Workshop on Unsupervised and Transfer Learning* (2012), pp. 37–49
80. H.O.A. Ahmed, M.D. Wong, A.K. Nandi, Intelligent condition monitoring method for bearing faults from highly compressed measurements using sparse over-complete features. Mech. Syst. Signal Process. **99**, 459–477 (2018)
81. C. Blum, D. Merkle, Swarm intelligence, in *Swarm Intelligence in Optimization*, ed. by C. Blum, D. Merkle (Springer, Boston, MA, 2008), pp. 43–85
82. A.E. Hassanien, E. Emary, *Swarm Intelligence: Principles, Advances, and Applications* (CRC Press, London, 2018)
83. X.S. Yang, Z. Cui, R. Xiao, A.H. Gandomi, M. Karamanoglu, (eds.), Swarm intelligence and bio-inspired computation: theory and applications, in *Newnes*, (2013)
84. R.C. Eberhart, Y. Shi, J. Kennedy, *Swarm Intelligence* (Elsevier, Amsterdam, 2001)
85. D. Karaboga, B. Basturk, A powerful and efficient algorithm for numerical function optimization: Artificial bee colony (ABC) algorithm. J. Global Optim. **39**(3), 459–471 (2007)
86. D. Karaboga, B. Basturk, On the performance of artificial bee colony (ABC) algorithm. Appl. Soft Comput. **8**(1), 687–697 (2008)
87. D. Karaboga, B. Gorkemli, C. Ozturk, N. Karaboga, A comprehensive survey: artificial bee colony (ABC) algorithm and applications. Artif. Intell. Rev. **42**(1), 21–57 (2014)
88. D. Karaboga, Artificial bee colony algorithm. Scholarpedia **5**(3), 6915 (2010)
89. U. Kose, A. Arslan, On the idea of a new artificial intelligence based optimization algorithm inspired from the nature of vortex. BRAIN. Broad Res. Artif. Intell. Neurosci. **5**(1–4), 60–66 (2015)

90. U. Kose, Development of Artificial Intelligence Based Optimization Algorithms (In Turkish), Doctoral dissertation, Selçuk University, Institute of Natural Sciences, (Konya, Turkey, 2017)
91. U. Kose, A. Arslan, Forecasting chaotic time series via anfis supported by vortex optimization algorithm: Applications on electroencephalogram time series. Arab. J. Sci. Eng. **42**(8), 3103–3114 (2017)
92. X.S. Yang, S. Deb, Cuckoo search via Lévy flights, in *2009 World Congress on Nature & Biologically Inspired Computing (NaBIC)* (IEEE, 2009), pp 210–214
93. P. Civicioglu, E. Besdok, A conceptual comparison of the Cuckoo-search, particle swarm optimization, differential evolution and artificial bee colony algorithms. Artif. Intell. Rev. **39**(4), 315–346 (2013)
94. Z. Cheng, R. Savit, Fractal and nonfractal behavior in Levy flights. J. Math. Phys. **28**(3), 592–597 (1987)
95. X. S. Yang, S. Deb, Engineering optimisation by cuckoo search. Int. J. Math. Modell. Numer. Optim. **1**(4), 330–343 (2010)
96. X.S. Yang, S. Deb, Cuckoo search: recent advances and applications. Neural Comput. Appl. **24**(1), 169–174 (2014)
97. S. Mirjalili, The ant lion optimizer. Adv. Eng. Softw. **83**, 80–98 (2015)
98. S. Mirjalili, P. Jangir, S. Saremi, Multi-objective ant lion optimizer: a multi-objective optimization algorithm for solving engineering problems. Appl. Intell. **46**(1), 79–95 (2017)
99. A.A. Heidari, H. Faris, S. Mirjalili, I. Aljarah, M. Mafarja, Ant Lion optimizer: theory, literature review, and application in multi-layer perceptron neural networks, in *Nature-Inspired Optimizers*. (Springer, Cham, 2020), pp. 23–46
100. A. Tabari, A. Ahmad, A new optimization method: electro-search algorithm. Comput. Chem. Eng. **103**, 1–11 (2017)
101. C. Blake, C. Merz, UCI repository of machine learning databases, Department of Information and Computer Science (University of California, Irvine, CA, USA, 1998). (Online). http://www.archive.ics.uci.edu/ml (2015)
102. Y. Chauvin, D.E. Rumelhart, *Backpropagation: Theory, Architectures, and Applications* (Psychology Press, 2013)
103. R. Hecht-Nielsen, Theory of the backpropagation neural network, in *Neural Networks for Perception*. (Academic Press, London, 1992), pp. 65–93
104. J.S. Jang, Self-learning fuzzy controllers based on temporal backpropagation. IEEE Trans. Neural Networks **3**(5), 714–723 (1992)
105. J.S. Jang, ANFIS: adaptive-network-based fuzzy inference system. IEEE Trans. Syst. Man Cybern. **23**(3), 665–685 (1993)
106. B. Scholkopf, A.J. Smola, *Learning with Kernels: Support Vector Machines, Regularization, Optimization, and Beyond* (MIT Press, Cambridge, MA, 2001)
107. N. Cristianini, J. Shawe-Taylor, *An Introduction to Support Vector Machines and Other Kernel-Based Learning Methods* (Cambridge University Press, Cambridge, 2000)
108. D.T. Larose, C.D. Larose, *K-nearest neighbor algorithm, in Discovering Knowledge in Data: An Introduction to Data Mining* (Wiley, New York, 2005), pp. 149–164
109. Z. Song, N. Roussopoulos, K-nearest neighbor search for moving query point, in *International Symposium on Spatial and Temporal Databases*. (Springer, Berlin, Heidelberg, 2001), pp. 79–96
110. J. Kennedy, *Swarm intelligence, in Handbook of Nature-Inspired and Innovative Computing* (Springer, Boston, MA, 2006), pp. 187–219
111. G. Beni, J. Wang, Swarm intelligence in cellular robotic systems, *Robots and Biological Systems: Towards a New Bionics?* (Springer, Berlin, Heidelberg, 1993), pp. 703–712
112. M.G. Hinchey, R. Sterritt, C. Rouff, Swarms and swarm intelligence. Computer **40**(4), 111–113 (2007)
113. A. Abraham, C. Grosan, V. Ramos (eds.), *Swarm Intelligence in Data Mining*, vol. 34 (Springer, Berlin, Heidelberg, 2007)
114. J.C. Bansal, P.K. Singh, N.R. Pal (eds.), *Evolutionary and Swarm Intelligence Algorithms* (Springer, Berlin, Heidelberg, 2019)

115. R.S. Parpinelli, G. Plichoski, R.S. Da Silva, P.H. Narloch, A review of techniques for online control of parameters in swarm intelligence and evolutionary computation algorithms. IJBIC **13**(1), 1–20 (2019)
116. X. Li, M. Clerc, Swarm intelligence, *Handbook of Metaheuristics* (Springer, Cham, 2019), pp. 353–384
117. B. Inje, S. Kumar, A. Nayyar, Swarm intelligence and evolutionary algorithms in disease diagnosis—introductory Aspects, in *Swarm Intelligence and Evolutionary Algorithms in Healthcare and Drug Development*. (Chapman and Hall/CRC, 2019), pp. 1–18
118. J. Del Ser, E. Villar, E. Osaba, Swarm Intelligence-Recent Advances, New Perspectives and Applications. (InTechOpen, 2019)
119. G.R. Raidl, J. Puchinger, C. Blum, Metaheuristic hybrids, *Handbook of Metaheuristics* (Springer, Cham, 2019), pp. 385–417
120. K. Kumar, J.P. Davim, *Optimization Using Evolutionary Algorithms and Metaheuristics: Applications in Engineering* (CRC Press, Boca Raton, FL, 2019)
121. H. Tavakoli, B.D. Barkdoll, Sustainability-based optimization algorithm. Int. J. Environ. Sci. Technol. **17**(3), 1537–1550 (2020)
122. T. Dede, M. Grzywiński, R.V. Rao, Jaya: a new meta-heuristic algorithm for the optimization of braced dome structures, *Advanced Engineering Optimization Through Intelligent Techniques* (Springer, Singapore, 2020), pp. 13–20
123. M. Mafarja, A.A. Heidari, H. Faris, S. Mirjalili, I. Aljarah, Dragonfly algorithm: theory, literature review, and application in feature selection, *Nature-Inspired Optimizers* (Springer, Cham, 2020), pp. 47–67
124. M.H. Sulaiman, Z. Mustaffa, M.M. Saari, H. Daniyal, Barnacles mating optimizer: a new bio-inspired algorithm for solving engineering optimization problems. Eng. Appl. Artif. Intell. **87**, 103330 (2020)
125. Y. Zhang, Z. Jin, Group teaching optimization algorithm: a novel metaheuristic method for solving global optimization problems. Expert Syst. Appl. **148**, 113246 (2020)
126. X. Zhong, D. Enke, Predicting the daily return direction of the stock market using hybrid machine learning algorithms. Fin. Innovation **5**(1), 4 (2019)
127. S. Ardabili, A. Mosavi, A.R. Várkonyi-Kóczy, Advances in machine learning modeling reviewing hybrid and ensemble methods, in *International Conference on Global Research and Education*. (Springer, Cham, 2019), pp. 215–227
128. T. Ma, C. Antoniou, T. Toledo, Hybrid machine learning algorithm and statistical time series model for network-wide traffic forecast. Transp. Res. Part C Emerg. Technol. **111**, 352–372 (2020)
129. S.N. Kumar, A.L. Fred, H.A. Kumar, P.S. Varghese, S.A. Jacob, Segmentation of anomalies in abdomen CT images by convolution neural network and classification by fuzzy support vector machine, *Hybrid Machine Intelligence for Medical Image Analysis* (Springer, Singapore, 2020), pp. 157–196
130. S. Bhattacharyya, D. Konar, J. Platos, C. Kar, K. Sharma (eds.), *Hybrid Machine Intelligence for Medical Image Analysis* (Springer, Singapore, 2020)
131. H.S. Shon, E. Batbaatar, K.O. Kim, E.J. Cha, K.A. Kim, Classification of kidney cancer data using cost-sensitive hybrid deep learning approach. Symmetry **12**(1), 154 (2020)
132. A. Shikalgar, S. Sonavane, Hybrid deep learning approach for classifying alzheimer disease based on multimodal data, *Computing in Engineering and Technology* (Springer, Singapore, 2020), pp. 511–520
133. N.B. Khulenjani, M.S. Abadeh, A hybrid feature selection and deep learning algorithm for cancer disease classification. Int. J. Comput. Inf. Eng. **14**(2), 55–59 (2020)
134. J. Lee, Y.K. Kim, A. Ha, S. Sun, Y.W. Kim, J.S. Kim, …, K.H. Park, Macular Ganglion cell-inner plexiform layer thickness prediction from Red-free fundus photography using. Hybrid deep learning model. Sci. Rep. **10**(1), 1–10 (2020)

Chapter 8
Psychological Personal Support System with Long Short Term Memory and Facial Expressions Recognition Approach

Advanced technologies for processing data gathered from the real world are widely used for improving tasks in different fields of the life. After especially rise of computer and communication technologies, it has been important to process the data rapidly and reach to automated decisions for making some tasks more practical in the digital world. Today, the raw data from the real world is easily processed by especially deep learning techniques [1–5]. It is remarkable that intelligent systems designed and developed thanks to deep learning can also be supported with some additional processing techniques in the context of data mining [6, 7] and image processing [8, 9]. Because it is important to analyze still images or live videos from the real world for making works of intelligent systems easier, image processing techniques are often used within intelligent systems. Here, typical applications include object detection, medical diagnosis, and facial recognition [10–14]. In the context of the real world, object detection is too important for understanding dynamic events, improving security, and even performing medical diagnosis for especially cancer and critical diseases requiring medical image analysis [15–18]. Among them, facial recognition is one of most remarkable research ways that is widely followed by researchers recently. It has become important especially when it was figured out that the data from people are key for understanding about their nature and interests. In even medical field, that research is a key point for psychological works and figuring out some signs of brain-oriented problems [19–21].

Among all the applications of image processing, facial recognition has received a great popularity in especially recent years [22–27]. Because facial recognition can open the doors to understanding automatically about people's emotions and possible actions-behaviors, hybrid systems of image processing and deep learning have been often used in different problem scopes [28–31]. On the other hand, in terms of target fields, the medical has a critical research ground, too. In medical, it is important to derive ideas about people's emotional state and feelings, in order to derive some psychological diagnosis and support people with depression, anxiety or any other psychological problems. By doing that, it can also be possible to predict more about

© The Editor(s) (if applicable) and The Author(s), under exclusive license to Springer Nature Singapore Pte Ltd. 2021
U. Kose et al., *Deep Learning for Medical Decision Support Systems*,
Studies in Computational Intelligence 909,
https://doi.org/10.1007/978-981-15-6325-6_8

neurological issues or diseases so that immediate actions for treatment can be taken accordingly.

Based on the explanations so far, this chapter introduces a typical use of deep learning and facial expression detection approach for ensuring a psychological personal support system, which can perform some analyzes with question-answer period or image-viewing session, in order to get some idea about emotional changes shown by the target person. The system can detect the person's instant emotion level and predict the possible psychological issues. In order to achieve that, a combination of image processing for facial recognition and a long short term memory (LSTM) are employed. At this point, facial recognition was used for understanding about each person's facial expressions instantly. In detail, a simple cam, which is appropriate enough to analyze facial expressions, is used to derive facial values and by adding some other different parameters to facial values, a set of data for predicting what to do ask next is formed as input to the deep learning model.

8.1   Background

The psychological personal support solution developed in this chapter is briefly based on two essential subjects: facial recognition and deep learning. Thanks to facial recognition, it was aimed to gather some instant data about emotional state. In order to do that, facial expressions associated with the facial recognition were detected. After that, it was aimed to feed the deep learning technique for making further decisions about which questions to be asked and/or which visual component to be shown to the target person. For deep learning purpose, a model of long short term memory (LSTM) was run as an effective tool.

8.1.1   Facial Recognition and Facial Expressions

Facial recognition is briefly measuring facial motion, which can be also used for understanding the target person's emotions [32]. Thanks to 43 muscles over our face, it is possible to produce around 10.000 different facial expressions [33]. Except from the physical features we observe, face and the expressions are important components for communication between two people and understanding enough about emotions of any future behavior that may be shown [34, 35]. Moving from these facts, it can be said that facial recognition is useful for physiology and any other fields it is associated with. In detail, especially marketing has a remarkable place among the studies regarding facial recognition. Because thanks to facial recognition, it is possible to understand about [36, 37]:

- Instant emotions shown by the person,
- The target person's physiological state,

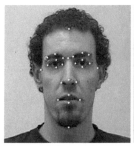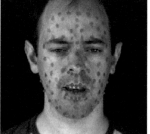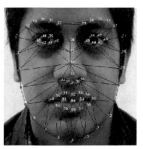

Fig. 8.1 Facial recognition done with computer-based systems [38–40]

- The target person's future behaviors-interests,
- The target person's instant attention state.

Since, the humankind is just able to understand emotions from some certain appearance of facial experiences, computer-based systems have been effective enough to give more detailed data by tracking certain points over faces. In this context, Fig. 8.1 shows some views from facial recognition done by computer-based systems [38–40].

As general, facial recognition may differ according to points detected over the face and also these points may be used for different purposes by using them as some kind of prediction data within machine learning techniques.

8.1.2 Long Short Term Memory

As the deep learning is the most important, advanced form the machine learning nowadays, there is an increasing diversity of different neural network models to be used for real-world problems. In this study, an important deep learning technique with its unique and interesting problem solution strategies has been used in the context of the developed support system. It is called as the long short term memory as a reference to its memory oriented features.

Long short term memory (LSTM) is briefly a recurrent neural network (RNN) architecture type so that it includes feedback connections rather than direct, one-way connections among artificial neurons. As a typical deep learning technique, LSTM is able to deal with sequences of data [41–43]. In typical running of long short term memory models, different neurons—components such as cell, output gate, input gate, and forget gate are all used accordingly. Here, a cell can remember the values over arbitrary time intervals and the other three neurons (gates) has the responsibility to regulate the information flow towards and from the cell. LSTM is a result of eliminating the exploding and vanishing gradient problems seen during training phases of RNN [44, 45]. Figure 8.2 shows a typical model of the LSTM [46, 47].

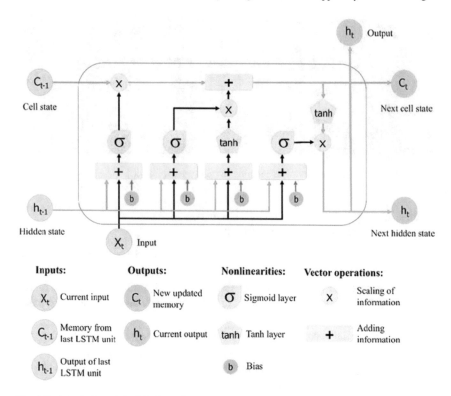

Fig. 8.2 A typical model of the long short term memory (LSTM) [46, 47]

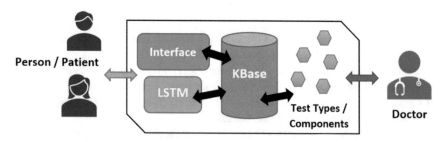

Fig. 8.3 General structure of the developed psychological personal support system

8.2 The Model of the Psychological Personal Support System

By considering the set-up of image processing and the LSTM explained under the previous section, the study here aimed to ensure an effective model for psychological personal support (Fig. 8.3). The following paragraphs briefly explain the employed components:

8.2.1   Infrastructure for Facial Expressions

The approach for facial recognition and understanding about emotions was used as a combination of ready infrastructure, which was developed in a previous study in [48] and further improved in this study. In the previous study, a system of detecting facial points and the emotions by moving from the learned facial points (recognition) was developed accordingly. Briefly, the 'detection infrastructure' here includes partially a trained data thanks to the following data sets [48–51]:

- **Data Set 1**: 490 photos with genders, and a total of 7 emotions,
- **Data Set 2**: Chicago data set, which employs 810 photos with genders, races, and a total of 7 emotions,
- **Data Set 3**: 100 photos chosen randomly by Boz and Kose [48].

The related infrastructure for accurate facial recognition and deriving emotions from facial expressions was obtained before by using all three data sets. In this study, it was improved by using live videos from a total of 30 different people. Here, a ready model of LSTM was fed via Microsoft Kinect 3D camera in order to get 3D face points and store detected emotions. In the associated literature, Microsoft Kinect 3D was often reported as an effective tool for recognition purposes [52–54]. By considering 30 different people, a total of 210 photos (by considering 7 emotions for each person) were used for improving the 'detection infrastructure' (Fig. 8.4). It is important that the system of emotion detection here considers 7 different emotions as 'fearful', 'angry', 'disgusted', 'surprised', 'happy', 'sad', and 'neutral'. By coding each emotion from 1 to 7, the detection infrastructure included detection data associated with x and y coordinates of 70 facial points, gender, race (if applicable) information, and also age information as the trained data for the LSTM model, which is responsible for making decisions on next test type/component. At this point, the model was fed by only percentages for each emotion, as given outputs by the ready detection infrastructure, which was trained with a total of almost 360 data rows of emotion detections.

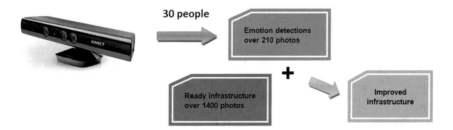

Fig. 8.4 Detection infrastructure

8.2.2 Long Short Term Memory Based Approach for Psychological Testing Process

The psychological support approach developed in this study is for running tests for understanding the psychological state of the person interacting with the system. The used LSTM model uses inputs for the face points, (and the other information such as gender, age, if used) for each emotion level, and also additional inputs determined by the doctor by considering i.e. following data gathered from the person during the test:

- Mental state grades,
- Level values for multiple intelligences
- Completion percentage of previously viewed test types,
- Responses given to the last asked question by the system,
- *Many more alternative data to be determined by the doctor.*

As it can be understood, the LSTM model input-output balance is determined adaptively according to the adjustments done by the doctor. On the other hand, there are three outputs as 'test type', 'emotion level', and 'selection border'. These outputs can be defined-explained as follows:

- **Test Type**: The test type is defined via numbers such as 1: only question, 2: visually supported text, 3: still visual, 4: animation, 5: music-sound, 6: video, … etc., which can be increased-decreased in time.
- **Emotion Level**: After getting instant face point states by the person, that output determines the level of emotion intensity. By considering a scale of [10, 100] (which may be also adjusted), less values cause less mixture of different emotional states whereas more values corresponds to more emotionally interactive test type to be provided next. Here, if the person seems sad, the emotion level may be higher in order to provide something asking and/or trying to figure out the exact psychological issue, and also making the person more comfortable or at least be leaving the sadness mood.
- **Selection Border**: By meeting with different content type and emotion level, the target test type to be processes next for the person can be determined according to selection border, which means the starting point to filter the whole material pool. For example, a value of 70 for selection border allows the system not to choose any test type having selection point less than 70. As it can be understood, each material in the system is also set with a selection point. Same and/or near selection point by different test types causes random selections.

In the context of the study here, the related network model has been trained by using sample data prepared synthetically by a total of 12 doctors working on mental issue states such as depression, anxiety, and also facial signs of serios neurological problems. Based on a total of 451 test types, a training and test data set was created accordingly. By considering different possible mental test grades, levels of multiple intelligences, any other numerical data as well as emotion levels for the people taking part over the system, and performing a data cleaning process for getting an accurate total number, a total of 3000 data rows was created. Here, 70% of the data (2100 data rows) was used for training while the rest of the 900-row data (30%) was used for testing the trained system. After 50 independent runs of the LSTM model, it was seen that the average accuracy of the model for the test data was 95.4%, which seems acceptable to run the system in real manner (for further evaluation).

In terms of a software approach, the system is briefly like an expert system [55–57], which is a method of artificial intelligence, as using the expert knowledge on the background for providing an interactive decision support and problem solution environment. The system here just starts asking questions to the person and considers different types of tests/components according to the given answers and the emotional expression detected by the person's face. Table 8.1 provides some examples of test types/components and the asked questions in the developed system.

The whole support system was designed and developed by considering object-oriented programming principles for fast and flexible enough coding infrastructure, which also has some simple functions for allowing integration with different upper-level software systems over an API based communication channel.

8.2.3   API Mechanism

The software based system of the psychological personal support system has been designed in the context of a module structure, which can communicate with upper-level software system that may be developed for a general purpose (That means the system here can be integrated into different upper-level software systems with an API mechanism, if they are appropriate enough to communicate). Whether it is coded via C oriented web programming languages or within other environments, main functions of the system have been developed by considering the following function definitions (the code definitions were made by eliminating detail syntax for specific languages):

- **PSS.define_input(free_index, value, connection)**: That function is used for taking an evaluation-task value from the upper-level software system, in order to feed the LSTM model by using any free input (if there is not any, then it may be created automatically) and the associated database connection details of the software system.
- **PSS.receive_directive(model_index)**: It is used for running the psychological personal support system and get the output(s) as returned value(s).
- **PSS.update_machine([input_values], TT, EL, SB)**: That function is used for defining a new test type/component by considering its values (according to the used model inputs, as in the form of a matrix) and the related TT: test type, EL: emotion level, and SB: selection border criteria values from the upper-level software system.

Table 8.1 Some examples of test types/components and the asked questions in the developed psychological personal support system

Test type	Example components	Example questions
Survey	Likert scale statements; multi-choice statements	*"Do you want to learn about your multiple intelligences?"* *"Do you want to take a survey about social life?"* *"Please fill the survey for what you feel about your job"*
Question-answer based	Emotional states; open questions	*"How do you feel today?"* *"Does that feeling make you comfortable?"* *"You look disgusted. Do you feel ill?"* *"You look sad. Do you feel lonely?"*
Music based	Emotional states; multi-choice statements; sound files	*"Please choose the best option explaining your happiness"* *"Do you want to listen to some melodies?"* *"Please tell me what you will feel after hearing the short-melody next"* *"Which type of music is appropriate for your current mood?"* *"You seem bored. Do you want to get some energic sound?"*
Video-music based	Emotional states; multi-choice statements	*"Please tell me what will you feel about the video next"* *"What do you feel about the boy in that video?"* *"Which scenario do you choose in the state shown at the video?"*
Animation-try based	Likert scale statements; emotional states; multi-choice statements; drawing	*"Please draw a shape over the area"* *"Which option does better explain your drawing?"* *"Please tell me about what did you feel about the animation you just watched"*

(continued)

Table 8.1 (continued)

Test type	Example components	Example questions
Visual image based	Emotional states; rorschach test images; shapes; photos	*"You feel sad today. Please tell me what do you see in the next image"* *"Which of the next images make you happy?"* *"Please choose the photos best describing your current mood"*
Visual image and question-answer based	Rorschach test images; shapes; photos; emotional states; open questions	*"How do you feel today?"* *"Do you feel tired now?"* *"Did you get up late today?"* *"Which color would you paint that house?"* *"Please tell me about the photo you will just see"*

- **PSS.gather_data(connection, [source_values], [target_values])**: That is used for gathering some data of test types from the database of the running upper-level software and then storing them into training database of the psychological personal support system, for automatically adapting the traditional using features of the upper-level software system to the psychological personal support approach.
- **PSS.evaluate(template_model, [content_type, TT, EL, SB]])**: It is used for running a reverse engineering over the stored content of the upper-level software system, in order to give idea about which emotion types-levels and test types may be needed for re-defining the related test component within the psychological personal support system. In order to achieve that, some predefined template LSTM models are used accordingly.

8.3 Evaluation

In order to evaluate the effectiveness of the developed system, which is combining detected emotions and additional tasks to determine what to show for target person, it was used three-month period by 12 doctors whose expertise is psychiatry. In detail, the doctors evaluated test processes for a total of 211 people. The system was trained thanks to the emotional/facial recognition data as well as psychological test flow data and the components provided by the doctors. After using period, the doctors were wanted to give some feedback comments regarding their experience on using the system. Some of the remarkable comments are as follows:

- *"This system detects the psychological diseases—problems correctly."*
- *"That's an easy-to-use, fast system that can be used for automatically diagnosing people's psychological problems."*

- *"Thanks to the system, my works have become easier to complete."*
- *"The system seems asking true questions for diagnosing an exact psychological state for the target people."*
- *"That system may be improved with additional features to be used for general purposes of medicine treatments of psychological diseases."*
- *"I want to continue to use that system."*

As evaluating the performance of the LSTM technique, an accuracy analysis was also done for different combinations of the gathered 3000-row data. As the accuracy is calculated according to the true detections of the target psychological issues mentioned by the doctors for each different input, each different combination of training/testing data included 70–30% training-test balance but with different test types/components included within them. Table 8.2 represents details regarding different data combination and the findings for success accuracies.

As it can be seen, the related LSTM infrastructure gets high accuracies for different combinations of the related data, by considering different psychological problem, as determined by the doctors. More diversity in the data as well as the target disease may cause reduce in the accuracy but it may be solved with additional data to train the LSTM model.

Table 8.2 Findings for different data combination and the findings for success accuracies

Combination No.	Test types in the combination	Target disease(s)	Data rows	Accuracy (%)
1	Likert scale statements; open questions; multi-choice statements	Depression	1090	88.60
2	Emotional states; multi-choice statements; rorschach test images; shapes	Personality disorders	2056	93.65
3	Multi-choice statements; sound files; multi-choice statements; drawing	Serious neurological	653	83.40
4	Emotional states; multi-choice statements	Anxiety	1981	95.25
5	Likert scale statements; multi-choice statements; drawing	Schizophrenia	418	84.55
6	Likert scale statements; photos	Dipolar disorder	1587	91.72

Thanks to both experience and technical based evaluations, it can be said that the psychological personal support system developed within this study seems effective enough to meet with the desired medical outcomes and the support in terms of decision making.

8.4 Results and Discussion

In this chapter, a psychological personal support system design was introduced as a hybrid formation of both image processing based facial recognition and also long short term memory (LSTM) as the deep learning infrastructure. In detail, a person's facial expressions were used as inputs to the LSTM model, with also alternative data, which may be effective for the system to decide what to ask/show-bring next, in order to determine psychological states about the target person. At this point, it is important that the solution design was thought as a typical decision-making/support mechanism that can be used as even API for integrating it to the upper-level software systems. The system developed here can use data regarding facial expressions (derived via facial recognition) and also alternative data (i.e. mental grades, completion rate of the previous tests, numerical data from alternative works over the upper-level software system) done by the person evaluated. The developed solution approach was evaluated by including it in process of different tests and 12 doctors were asked to provide their feedback about the decisions made by the system. Also, the accuracy rate of the system was evaluated in terms of different combinations of the provided data for training and the testing. According to the findings, the system seems successful enough on ensuring psychological decisions and giving appropriate enough support in this manner.

In the future, it is also possible to improve such system with additional adjustments. For example, the deep learning infrastructure can be analyzed for further revisions to improve the performance and getting better decision-making. That can be done by adjusting parameters of the LSTM or replacing it with different deep learning techniques. It is also possible to compare the current system with some other deep leaning techniques i.e. convolutional neural network (CNN), or deep belief networks or known traditional machine learning techniques such as decision trees, support vector machines, multi-layer artificial neural network or extreme learning machine, for understanding if the system can be improved more. On the other hand, the developed solution design of applying tests/ensuring question-answer processes can be continued to be evaluated by applying it in different cases and target people groups. Finally, the system may also be supported with more biometric data from people, in order to see if it is possible to learn more about instant emotional state with alternative data.

8.5 Summary

Because today's life causes many people to experience psychological problems in general, it has become a need to see doctors for further discussing about details of the problems and figuring out how to deal with and treat them. Such situations always require careful evaluation generally done by asking questions and trying to understand psychological state, mood and emotions about the target person. As people's faces also give important signs, it can be possible to track facial expressions and follow an emotion supported, intelligent support process, by considering combinations of different tests and emotions at the one hand. In this chapter, use of facial recognition and deep learning was explained in the context of a psychological personal support system. The system used a specific, remarkable deep learning technique: long short term memory (LSTM) in order to achieve an automated approach of diagnosis and prediction of next tests/components to be shown. Additionally, the system here has been responsible for directing to whole test process applied for a person to understand accurately about problems. The evaluation works show positive results in terms of personal usage experiences by the doctors and the detection accuracy of the LSTM model.

The future of the medical decision support systems seems based on different software systems including use of artificial intelligence/deep learning for diagnosing specific disease including psychological ones. Except from diagnosis of physical and metabolic diseases, research works for developing intelligent systems considering psychological problems have still open problems and further innovations to be done so that the associated literature will be expanding to that direction, too.

8.6 Further Learning

For learning more about psychology, psychiatry, and neurology-oriented research works with artificial intelligence, machine/deep learning, the interested readers are referred to [58–67].

In order to understand deeper about recent uses of the long short term memory (LSTM), readers can examine [68–76].

For more about alternative, very recent works on facial recognition and emotional detection, the readers can read [77–84].

References

1. I. Goodfellow, Y. Bengio, A. Courville, *Deep Learning* (MIT Press, 2016)
2. A. Gulli, S. Pal, *Deep Learning with Keras* (Packt Publishing Ltd, 2017)
3. N. Buduma, N. Locascio, *Fundamentals of Deep Learning: Designing Next-Generation Machine Intelligence Algorithms.* (O'Reilly Media, Inc., 2017)

4. S.K. Zhou, H. Greenspan, D. Shen, eds. *Deep Learning for Medical Image Analysis* (Academic Press, 2017)
5. M. Fullan, J. Quinn, J. McEachen, *Deep Learning: Engage the World Change the World* (Corwin Press, 2017)
6. C.C. Aggarwal, *Data Mining: The Textbook* (Springer, 2015)
7. I.H. Witten, E. Frank, M.A. Hall, C.J. Pal, *Data Mining: Practical Machine Learning Tools and Techniques* (Morgan Kaufmann, 2016)
8. A.C. Bovik, *Handbook of Image and Video Processing* (Academic Press, 2010)
9. J.C. Russ, *The Image Processing Handbook* (CRC Press, 2016)
10. E. Alpaydin, *Introduction to Machine Learning* (MIT Press, 2009)
11. T.O. Ayodele, *Introduction to Machine Learning* (INTECH Open Access Publisher, 2010)
12. S. Marsland, *Machine Learning: An Algorithmic Perspective* (Chapman and Hall/CRC, 2014)
13. T.M. Mitchell, *The Discipline of Machine Learning*, vol. 9 (Carnegie Mellon University, School of Computer Science, Machine Learning Department, Pittsburgh, PA, 2006)
14. S. Mitra, S. Datta, T. Perkins, G. Michailidis, *Introduction to Machine Learning and Bioinformatics* (Chapman and Hall/CRC, 2008)
15. R. Cipolla, S. Battiato, G.M. Farinella, *Machine Learning for Computer Vision*, vol 5 (Springer, 2013)
16. J. Ponce, M. Hebert, C. Schmid, A. Zisserman, eds. *Toward Category-Level Object Recognition*, vol 4170 (Springer, 2007)
17. G. Shaogang, P. Alexandra, *Dynamic Vision: from Images to Face Recognition* (World Scientific, 2000)
18. S.K. Zhou, *Medical Image Recognition, Segmentation and Parsing: Machine Learning and Multiple Object Approaches* (Academic Press, 2015)
19. R. Adolphs, Recognizing emotion from facial expressions: psychological and neurological mechanisms. Behav. Cogn. Neurosci. Rev. **1**(1), 21–62.A (2002)
20. T.K. Shackelford, R.J. Larsen, Facial asymmetry as an indicator of psychological, emotional, and physiological distress. J. Pers. Soc. Psychol. **72**(2), 456 (1997)
21. J.P. Robinson, P.R. Shaver, L.S. Wrightsman, eds. *Measures of Personality and Social Psychological Attitudes: Measures of Social Psychological Attitudes*, vol 1 (Academic Press, 2013)
22. W. AbdAlmageed, Y. Wu, S. Rawls, S. Harel, T. Hassner, I., Masi, R. Nevatia, Face recognition using deep multi-pose representations, in *2016 IEEE Winter Conference on Applications of Computer Vision (WACV)*, pp. 1–9. IEEE
23. B. Amos, B. Ludwiczuk, M. Satyanarayanan, Openface: a general-purpose face recognition library with mobile applications. CMU Sch. Comput. Sci. (2016)
24. C. Ding, D. Tao, Trunk-branch ensemble convolutional neural networks for video-based face recognition. IEEE Trans. Pattern Anal. Mach. Intell. (2017)
25. P. Karczmarek, A. Kiersztyn, W. Pedrycz, An evaluation of fuzzy measure for face recognition, in *International Conference on Artificial Intelligence and Soft Computing* (Springer, Cham, 2017), pp. 668–676
26. A.T. Lopes, E. de Aguiar, A.F. De Souza, T. Oliveira-Santos, Facial expression recognition with convolutional neural networks: coping with few data and the training sample order. Pattern Recogn. **61**, 610–628 (2017)
27. Y.D. Zhang, Z.J. Yang, H.M. Lu, X.X. Zhou, P. Phillips, Q.M. Liu, S.H. Wang, Facial emotion recognition based on biorthogonal wavelet entropy, fuzzy support vector machine, and stratified cross validation. IEEE Access **4**, 8375–8385 (2016)
28. M.Z. Uddin, M.M. Hassan, A. Almogren, M. Zuair, G. Fortino, J. Torresen, A facial expression recognition system using robust face features from depth videos and deep learning. Comput. Electr. Eng. **63**, 114–125 (2017)
29. V. Mavani, S. Raman, K.P. Miyapuram, Facial expression recognition using visual saliency and deep learning, in *Proceedings of the IEEE International Conference on Computer Vision Workshops*, pp. 2783–2788 (2017)
30. N. Jain, S. Kumar, A. Kumar, P. Shamsolmoali, M. Zareapoor, Hybrid deep neural networks for face emotion recognition. Pattern Recogn. Lett. **115**, 101–106 (2018)

31. S. Zhang, X. Pan, Y. Cui, X. Zhao, L. Liu, Learning affective video features for facial expression recognition via hybrid deep learning. IEEE Access **7**, 32297–32304 (2019)
32. Y. Tian, T. Kanade, J.F. Cohn, Facial expression recognition, in *Handbook of Face Recognition* (Springer, London, 2011), pp. 487–519
33. A. Bejgu, I. Mocanu, Facial emotion recognition using Kinect. J. Inf. Syst. Oper. Manag. **1 (2014)**
34. P. Ekman, E.L. Rosenberg (eds.), *What the Face Reveals: Basic and Applied Studies of Spontaneous Expression Using the Facial Action Coding System (FACS)* (Oxford University Press, USA, 1997)
35. A. Kendon, Language and gesture: unity or duality, in *Language and Gesture: Window into Thought and Action* (Cambridge Unviersity Press, Cambridge, 2000)
36. A.K. Jain, S.Z. Li, *Handbook of Face Recognition* (Springer, New York, 2011)
37. H. Wechsler, J.P. Phillips, V. Bruce, F.F. Soulié, T.S. Huang, eds. *Face Recognition: From Theory to Applications*, vol 163 (Springer Science and Business Media, 2012)
38. S. Asadiabadi, R. Sadiq, E. Erzin, Multimodal speech driven facial shape animation using deep neural networks, in *2018 Asia-Pacific Signal and Information Processing Association Annual Summit and Conference (APSIPA ASC)*, pp. 1508–1512, IEEE (2018)
39. A. Gera, A. Bhattacharya, Emotion recognition from audio and visual data using f-score based fusion, in *Proceedings of the 1st IKDD Conference on Data Sciences* (ACM, 2014), pp. 1–10
40. Y. Tie, L. Guan, Automatic landmark point detection and tracking for human facial expressions. EURASIP J. Image Video Process. **2013**(1), 8 (2013)
41. S. Hochreiter, J. Schmidhuber, Long short-term memory. Neural Comput. **9**(8), 1735–1780 (1997)
42. H. Sak, A.W. Senior, F. Beaufays, Long short-term memory recurrent neural network architectures for large scale acoustic modeling (2014)
43. X. Zhu, P. Sobihani, H. Guo, Long short-term memory over recursive structures, in *International Conference on Machine Learning*, pp. 1604–1612 (2015)
44. A. Graves, Long short-term memory, in *Supervised Sequence Labelling with Recurrent Neural Networks* (Springer, Berlin, Heidelberg, 2012), pp. 37–45
45. Y. Zhang, G. Chen, D. Yu, K. Yaco, S. Khudanpur, J. Glass, Highway long short-term memory rnns for distant speech recognition, in *2016 IEEE International Conference on Acoustics, Speech and Signal Processing (ICASSP)*, pp. 5755–5759. IEEE (2016)
46. X.H. Le, H.V. Ho, G. Lee, S. Jung, Application of long short-term memory (LSTM) neural network for flood forecasting. Water **11**(7), 1387 (2019)
47. S. Yan, Understanding LSTM and Its Diagrams. Online: https://medium.com/mlreview/understanding-lstm-and-its-diagrams-37e2f46f1714. Retrieved 16 January 2020
48. H. Boz, U. Kose, Emotion Extraction from Facial Expressions by Using Artificial Intelligence Techniques. BRAIN: Broad Res. Artif. Intell. Neurosci. **9**(1), 5–16 (2018)
49. M. Grgic, K. Delac, Face Recognition Homepage. Online: http://www.face-rec.org/databases/. Retrieved 23 December 2017
50. R. Gross, Face databases, in *Handbook of Face Recognition*, eds. by S.Z. Stan, A.K. Jain (Springer, 2005)
51. D.S. Ma, J. Correll, B. Wittenbrink, The Chicago face database: a free stimulus set of faces and norming data. Behav. Res. Methods **47**(4), 1122–1135 (2015)
52. C. Cao, Y. Weng, S. Zhou, Y. Tong, K. Zhou, Facewarehouse: a 3d facial expression database for visual computing. IEEE Trans. Visual Comput. Graphics **20**(3), 413–425 (2014)
53. K. Sato, T. Nose, A. Ito, Y. Chiba, A. Ito, T. Shinozaki, A Study on 2D photo-realistic facial animation generation using 3D facial feature points and deep neural networks, in *International Conference on Intelligent Information Hiding and Multimedia Signal Processing* (Springer, Cham, 2017), pp. 112–118
54. E. Silverstein, M. Snyder, Implementation of facial recognition with Microsoft Kinect v2 sensor for patient verification. Med. Phys. **44**(6), 2391–2399 (2017)
55. J.C. Giarratano, G. Riley, *Expert Systems* (PWS Publishing Co, 1998)

56. P. Pandey, R. Litoriya, A predictive fuzzy expert system for crop disease diagnostic and decision support, in *Fuzzy Expert Systems and Applications in Agricultural Diagnosis* (IGI Global, 2020), pp. 175–194
57. S.R. Qwaider, S. S. Abu Naser, Expert system for diagnosing ankle diseases. Int. J. Eng. Inf. Syst. (IJEAIS) (2017)
58. D.B. Dwyer, P. Falkai, N. Koutsouleris, Machine learning approaches for clinical psychology and psychiatry. Annu. Rev. Clin. Psychol. **14**, 91–118 (2018)
59. D. Bone, M.S. Goodwin, M.P. Black, C.C. Lee, K. Audhkhasi, S. Narayanan, Applying machine learning to facilitate autism diagnostics: pitfalls and promises. J. Autism Dev. Disord. **45**(5), 1121–1136 (2015)
60. D. Bone, S.L. Bishop, M.P. Black, M.S. Goodwin, C. Lord, S.S. Narayanan, Use of machine learning to improve autism screening and diagnostic instruments: effectiveness, efficiency, and multi-instrument fusion. J. Child Psychol. Psychiatry **57**(8), 927–937 (2016)
61. K. Pancerz, O. Mich, A. Burda, J. Gomuła, A tool for computer-aided diagnosis of psychological disorders based on the MMPI test: an overview, in *Applications of Computational Intelligence in Biomedical Technology* (Springer, Cham, 2016), pp. 201–213
62. Z.S. Zheng, N. Reggente, E. Lutkenhoff, A.M. Owen, M.M. Monti, Disentangling disorders of consciousness: Insights from diffusion tensor imaging and machine learning. Hum. Brain Mapp. **38**(1), 431–443 (2017)
63. S. Mani, M.B. Dick, M. J. Pazzani, E. L. Teng, D. Kempler, I.M. Taussig, Refinement of neuro-psychological tests for dementia screening in a cross cultural population using machine learning, in *Joint European Conference on Artificial Intelligence in Medicine and Medical Decision Making* (Springer, Berlin, Heidelberg, 1999), pp. 326–335
64. R. Dinga, A.F. Marquand, D.J. Veltman, A.T. Beekman, R.A. Schoevers, A.M. van Hemert, L. Schmaal, Predicting the naturalistic course of depression from a wide range of clinical, psychological, and biological data: a machine learning approach. Transl. Psychiatry **8**(1), 1–11 (2018)
65. W. Liu, M. Li, L. Yi, Identifying children with autism spectrum disorder based on their face processing abnormality: a machine learning framework. Autism Res. **9**(8), 888–898 (2016)
66. W. Jarrold, B. Peintner, D. Wilkins, D. Vergryi, C. Richey, M.L. Gorno-Tempini, J. Ogar, Aided diagnosis of dementia type through computer-based analysis of spontaneous speech, in *Proceedings of the Workshop on Computational Linguistics and Clinical Psychology: From Linguistic Signal to Clinical Reality*, pp. 27–37 (2014)
67. A.B. Shatte, D.M. Hutchinson, S.J. Teague, Machine learning in mental health: a scoping review of methods and applications. Psychol. Med. **49**(9), 1426–1448 (2019)
68. T. Adler, M. Erhard, M. Krenn, J. Brandstetter, J. Kofler, S. Hochreiter, Quantum Optical Experiments Modeled by Long Short-Term Memory (2019). arXiv preprint arXiv:1910.13804
69. Y.Y. Hong, J.J.F. Martinez, A.C. Fajardo, Day-ahead solar irradiation forecasting utilizing gramian angular field and convolutional long short-term memory. IEEE Access **8**, 18741–18753 (2020)
70. A. Chandra, S.K. Khatri, Spam SMS filtering using recurrent neural network and long short term memory, in *2019 4th International Conference on Information Systems and Computer Networks (ISCON)* (IEEE, 2019), pp. 118–122
71. F. Wei, U.T. Nguyen, Twitter bot detection using bidirectional long short-term memory neural networks and word embeddings, in *2019 First IEEE International Conference on Trust, Privacy and Security in Intelligent Systems and Applications (TPS-ISA)* (IEEE, 2019), pp. 101–109
72. C. Li, Z. Wang, M. Rao, D. Belkin, W. Song, H. Jiang, N. Ge, Long short-term memory networks in memristor crossbar arrays. Nat. Mach. Intell. **1**(1), 49–57 (2019)
73. M. Al-Smadi, B. Talafha, M. Al-Ayyoub, Y. Jararweh, Using long short-term memory deep neural networks for aspect-based sentiment analysis of Arabic reviews. Int. J. Mach. Learn. Cybernet. **10**(8), 2163–2175 (2019)
74. S.R. de Assis Neto, G.L. Santos, E. da Silva Rocha, M. Bendechache, P. Rosati, T. Lynn, P.T. Endo, Detecting human activities based on a multimodal sensor data set using a bidirectional long short-term memory model: a case study, in *Challenges and Trends in Multimodal Fall Detection for Healthcare* (Springer, Cham, 2020), pp. 31–51

75. N. Somu, G.R. MR, K. Ramamritham, A hybrid model for building energy consumption forecasting using long short term memory networks. Appl. Energy **261**, 114131 (2020)
76. Z. Sun, C. Wang, Z. Ye, H. Bi, Long short-term memory network-based emission models for conventional and new energy buses. Int. J. Sustain. Transp. 1–10 (2020)
77. D.K. Jain, P. Shamsolmoali, P. Sehdev, Extended deep neural network for facial emotion recognition. Pattern Recogn. Lett. **120**, 69–74 (2019)
78. S. Passardi, P. Peyk, M. Rufer, T.S. Wingenbach, M.C. Pfaltz, Facial mimicry, facial emotion recognition and alexithymia in post-traumatic stress disorder. Behav. Res. Ther. **122**, 103436 (2019)
79. E. Dandıl, R. Özdemir, Real-time facial emotion classification using deep learning. Data Sci. Appl. **2**(1), 13–17 (2019)
80. R.K. Pandey, S. Karmakar, A.G. Ramakrishnan, N. Saha, Improving Facial Emotion Recognition Systems Using Gradient and Laplacian Images (2019). arXiv preprint arXiv:1902.05411
81. N. Ouherrou, O. Elhammoumi, F. Benmarrakchi, J. El Kafi, Comparative study on emotions analysis from facial expressions in children with and without learning disabilities in virtual learning environment. Educ. Inf. Technol. **24**(2), 1777–1792 (2019)
82. J. Deng, G. Pang, Z. Zhang, Z. Pang, H. Yang, G. Yang, cGAN based facial expression recognition for human-robot interaction. IEEE Access **7**, 9848–9859 (2019)
83. B. Lu, X. Duan, Facial expression recognition based on strengthened deep belief network with eye movements information, in *Artificial Intelligence in China* (Springer, Singapore, 2020), pp. 645–652
84. A. Lopez-Rincon, Emotion recognition using facial expressions in children using the NAO robot, in *2019 International Conference on Electronics, Communications and Computers (CONIELECOMP)* (IEEE, 2019), pp. 146–153

Chapter 9
Diagnosing of Diabetic Retinopathy with Image Dehazing and Capsule Network

As it was discussed before in Chap. 4, the disease of diabetic retinopathy (DR) ensure terrible results such as blindness, it has been a remarkable medical problem examined recently. Here, especially retinal pathologies can be the biggest problem for millions of blindness cases seen world-wide [1]. When all the cases of blindness are examined in detail, it was reported that there are around 2 million diabetic retinopathy cases causing the blindness so that early diagnosis has taken many steps away in terms of having the highest priority in eliminating or at least slowing down disease factors (causing blindness) and so that reducing the rates of blindness at the final [2, 3].

Considering Fig. 9.1, which is a more detailed view than the one provided in Chap. 4, it possible to see state of the retina with the components such as blood vessels, macula, and the optic disc. As changes over these components are signs of the DR, the disease can be examined in two stages such non-proliferative DR (NPDR) where diabetes causes damages over the blood vessels so that the blood affects function of the retina negatively, and the proliferative DR (PDR) where normal blood vessels grow over the retina and may cause to the blindness at the end. Here, NPDR can lead to different signs of retinopathy called as micro aneurysms (MAs), hard and soft exudates (EXs), hemorrhages (HMs), and the inter-retinal microvascular abnormalities (IRMA) [1, 4]. Gathering all signs-states into one hand, it is possible to talk about five-type DR, as show in Fig. 9.1 [5].

As recalled the diagnosis of DR, it is possible to briefly express some about alternative research works. Sreejini and Govindan have used optic disc elimination, exudate segmentation, fovea and macular region localization and then the classification of DR. In detail, they employed image processing, an intelligent optimization technique: Particle Swarm Optimization (PSO), and the Fuzzy C-Means Clustering [6]. Seoud and his colleagues proposed a grading system, which can automatically perform a decision-making approach for DR. In their study, they identified a red lesion to form a probability map regarding the lesion and then get a classification approach using 35 characteristics combining size as well as probability information [7]. Acharya et al. used a support vector machine model for mass screening of diabetic

© The Editor(s) (if applicable) and The Author(s), under exclusive license to Springer Nature Singapore Pte Ltd. 2021
U. Kose et al., *Deep Learning for Medical Decision Support Systems*,
Studies in Computational Intelligence 909,
https://doi.org/10.1007/978-981-15-6325-6_9

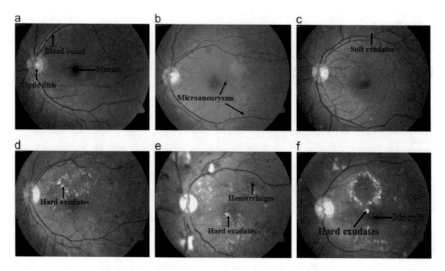

Fig. 9.1 Eye retina states in the context of DR: **a** Normal—**b** Mild NPDR—**c** Moderate NPDR—**d** Severe NPDR—**e** Prolific DR—**f** Macular edema [5]

retinopathy, which was done automatically via tissue properties [8]. In another study, Safitri and Juniati ensured an early detection of micro aneurysms (MA) by removing candidate sites for MAs within the retinal image, and then classifying the related regions with a hybrid approach including Gaussian mixing model and a model of support vector machine [9]. Savarkar and colleagues proposed a method of detecting MAs by analyzing density values along discrete segments of different directions centered in the candidate pixel. In this method, the peak values were determined first and then the feature set was determined and classified [10]. Finally, Akremetal et al. have a research of diagnosing DR, done with the fractal analysis, and the k-nearest neighbor (kNN) techniques [11].

In this chapter, the diagnosis of DR was solved that time with the Capsule Network, which is called also as CapsNet briefly. CapsNet is actually an improved version of the convolutional neural networks (CNN), which is a widely used deep learning technique, as employing important advantages of the deep learning [12]. In addition to the solution in Chap. 4, Deperlioglu and Kose used before a practical image processing method to improve retinal fundus images including HSV, V transformation algorithm and histogram equalization techniques for better classifying the images (diagnosis) with the CNN [13]. An alternative work with the CNN was also done in [14], by employing histogram equalization (HE) as well as the contrast limited adaptive histogram equalization (CLAHE) for providing better data for the CNN. Also, there is another alternative use of CNN and development of a diagnosis/decision support system with no user input, as done by Pratt et al. in [15]. Here, the question of if CapsNet can improve the results more against especially CNN was tried to be answered with also alternative use of image processing with a simple technique of image dehazing accordingly.

9.1 Materials and Method

In the study, the diagnosis of the DR was done with two-step approach including image processing and then classification with the CapsNet. For the training/tests, the Kaggle Diabetic Retinopathy Detection database was chosen as the target data in the study. The related stages in detail for the DR diagnosis are represented in Fig. 9.2.

9.1.1 Kaggle Diabetic Retinopathy Database for Diagnosis

The database of DR provided in the Kaggle platform is briefly a public set including over 80,000 colorful fundus images [16]. The first data set consisted of 88,702 colorful fundus images gathered from a total of 44,351 patients. Images were collected from several primary found centers in California and elsewhere with various digital fundus cameras. As all files in jpeg format, the definitions are respectively 433 × 289 pixels to 5184 × 3456 pixels (as the median definition: 3888 × 2592 pixels), and the related images were uploaded to the EyePACS, which is a DR screening platform [17]. For each eye, the severity of DR was rated by an expert on the ETDRS [18] scale. These are respectively 'absence-of DR', 'mild non-proliferative DR (NPDR)', 'moderate NPDR', 'severe NPDR' and 'proliferative DR (PDR) [19].

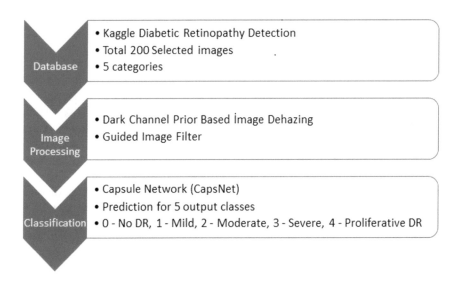

Fig. 9.2 The stages in detail for the diagnosis of the diabetic retinopathy

9.1.2 Image Processing

In this study, a simple and fast image enhancement method was used which gives close performance to mixed methods. This method consists of dark-channel prior based image dehazing, and also image guided filter.

The dark-channel prior based is a type of statistic for outdoors-free images image dehazing. It uses the approach of an important observation/most local patches on outdoor airless images include some pixels with a very low density in at least one-color channel. Just before, running that in the haze imaging model, the thickness of the haze and also obtaining of a high-quality haze-free image are possible to be directly predicted. The dark-channel prior here is just a simple but powerful enough prior, in order to be used for removal of single image haze. As a result of combining the haze imaging model with the prior, the removal of single image haze becomes more effective and in an easier form [20].

After dehazing, a guided filter is used for smoothing the colors and sharping the edges. The guided filter formed as from a local linear model ensures calculation of the filtering output, thanks to the contents of a grid image, which may be the input image itself or another different image. Here, it is possible to use the guided filter as an edge protector straightening operator, such as the popular bilateral filter, but has better behavior as close to the related edges. The guided filter can also transfer the structures of the orientation image to the filtering output so that it enables new filtering applications such as guided feathering and the dehazing [21].

9.1.3 Classification

The classification approach for diagnosing DR in this study was done with the Capsule Network (CapsNet), which is an effective, recent deep learning techniques. The CapsNet has been applied over the related Kaggle database accordingly, after the image processing phase.

CapsNet is a recent deep learning architecture employing capsules, which are groups of artificial neurons as the data processing components. CapsNet has been developed as a solution for the problem of discarding some information (i.e. position and the pose of the target object) because of the data routing process seen in convolutional neural networks (CNN). In a typical CapsNet, each capsule can determine a single component within the target object, and eventually, all capsules form the whole structure of the object collaboratively [22–24]. As a typical improvement of the CNN, CapsNet models include multi-layers. Figure 9.3 represents a typical structure of the CapsNet [25].

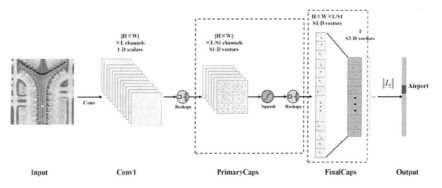

Fig. 9.3 A typical structure of the capsule network (CapsNet) [25]

9.1.4 Evaluation of the Diagnosis

As used in different medical applications including especially diagnosis, the following evaluation metrics were used in this study, for evaluating the developed solution [26]:

$$\text{Accuracy} = (\text{TrP} + \text{TrN})/N \tag{1}$$

$$\text{Sensitivity} = \text{TrP}/P \tag{2}$$

$$\text{Specificity} = \text{TrN}/N \tag{3}$$

$$\text{Precision} = \text{TrP}/(\text{TrP} + \text{FrP}) \tag{4}$$

$$\text{Recall} = \text{Sensitivity} \tag{5}$$

$$f\_score = 2 * [(\text{Precision} * \text{Recall})/(\text{Precision} + \text{Recall})] \tag{6}$$

$$\text{gmean} = \text{sqrt}(\text{Sensitivity} * \text{Specificity}) \tag{7}$$

In the context of the related equations, TrP and FrP mean respectively as the total number of true positive, and the total number of false positive regarding the performed diagnosis. Additionally, TrN and FrN correspond to the total number of true negative, and the total number of false negatives seen within the diagnosis N is for the total number of the data/samples, as meaning also sum of positives (P), and negatives (N). For a specific classification technique, precision of diagnosing correctly is associated with the ratio of accuracy. On the other hand, the Sensitivity is for defining the extent to which the classifier defines target class formation correctly, and the Specificity is for the separation capability for target classes [27, 28].

9.2 Application and Evaluation

MATLAB r2017a software was used in all image processing and the classification/diagnosis processes. In the study, 200 color fundus digital images in the Kaggle database were used to evaluate the performance of the image processing supporting CapsNet model. At this point, 200 images including 157 no DR (0), 10 mild NPDR (1), 27 moderate NPDR (2), 4 severe NPDR (3), and 2 proliferative DR (PDR) (4) were selected and used accordingly. Consequently, the output classes of the classification are five such as 0, 1, 2, 3, and 4.

First, image enhancement to these images was performed. Figure 9.4 shows the images after the image enhancement steps for 46_left.jpeg. In the image processing studies, entropy value and mean value were examined in order to evaluate the obtained results. For example, for the "46_left.jpeg" image, the entropy value of the original image measured is 2.2036. The Entropy value of the improved image increased to 2.6634. Similarly, the mean value regarding the original image is 204.2431. The mean value of the improved image has increased to 209.6221. Since higher entropy and mean values mean better visualization, there is improvement in images.

In order to better understand the improvements in the image, only original images and improved images are shown in Fig. 9.5.

In the context of the DR diagnosis process, the obtained colorful fundus images were classified by the CapsNet model. In order to design a model for diagnosing the DR, the CapsNet here consisted of 5 layers at total. These layers are respectively image input layer (with parameters of [195 322 3]), convolutional layer (3 × 3 × 256), primary caps (3 × 3 × (1 × 256)), fundus caps ((7 × 7) × 256), and the output layer (classification layer).

In the classification/diagnosis, 200 images from the Kaggle database were used while 80% of these images were for training, and the remaining 20% was for the test. For randomly selected training and test data, the classification process was repeated 20 times. The obtained findings in terms of the lowest-average-highest values for the performance evaluation metrics are given in Table 9.1.

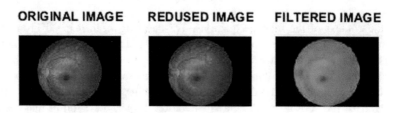

Fig. 9.4 The images after the image processing steps

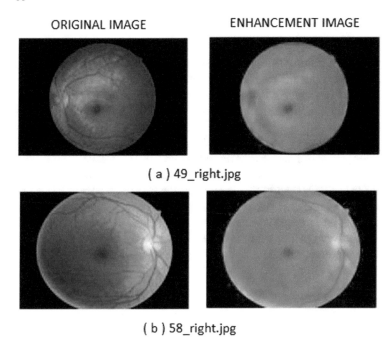

ORIGINAL IMAGE   ENHANCEMENT IMAGE

(a) 49_right.jpg

(b) 58_right.jpg

Fig. 9.5 Original images and improved images

Table 9.1 The lowest, the average and the highest values of performance metrics

Criteria	Lowest	Average	Highest
Accuracy	0.9225	0.9484	0.9650
Sensitivity	0.8150	0.8468	0.8800
Specificity	0.9650	0.9823	0.9833
Precision	0.8950	0.8468	0.8800
Recall	0.8150	0.8468	0.8800
F-score	0.8150	0.8468	0.8800
gmean	0.8143	0.8287	0.8406

As it is seen from the obtained findings the combination of the image dehazing and the CapsNet model has high values in terms of different evaluation metrics. That can be indicated that the diagnosis solution has a very high sampling, selection and estimation ability.

9.3 Results

In this chapter, it is aimed to explain an easy method instead of creating DR diagnostic methods by not using different heavy-detailed image processing methods and artificial intelligence techniques. In this context, easy diagnosis of diabetic retinopathy by defogging of the fundus image using a dark canal priority method and classification using capsule networks (CapsNet) have been proposed. In order to test the performance of the proposed method, an application was created with Kaggle Diabetic Retinopathy diagnosis database. After image processing, a classification study was performed with a CapsNet model. A total of 20 trials were performed and the average values of the criteria used in performance evaluation were taken. Obtained results show that the developed model a very high sampling, selection and estimation ability. Thus, the proposed method is very effective and efficient in the diagnosis of DR from retinal fundus images. For the future works different image processing method can be added or different variations of the CapsNet can also be implemented.

9.4 Summary

The humankind has always been dealing with serious disease needing early diagnosis for better treatment results at end. As the diabetic retinopathy (DR) has the potential of causing blindness, the associated literature of artificial intelligence has given a remarkable emphasis for designing diagnosis solutions, which has early diagnosis mechanism. In order to achieve that, image processing and machine/deep learning all have great synergy to develop innovative and robust solutions. As similar, this chapter provided an alternative solution combining image dehazing and the Capsule Network (CapsNet). The solution provided here is just another example of diagnosing DR, as explained before in Chap. 4, too. It can be clearly seen that there are open ways to derive alternative solutions for trying to improve obtained results. The solutions provided in both Chap. 4 and this chapter can also be applied for diagnosis of alternative diseases, which can be diagnosed from image data.

As the chapters past so far provided a general collection of medical decision support rising over diagnosis processes, there are still many more alternative research ways to be done, by considering the wide variety of diseases. Although the humankind desires a disease-free world, that seems impossible because of the chaos in the life and the nature itself. However, the future will be still associated with further developments and alternative solution ideas in the intersection of artificial intelligence and the field of medical. By considering deep learning and the topic of medical decision support systems, the final Chap. 10 is devoted to a general discussion on what kind of future may be shaped thanks to strong relation between deep learning-oriented decision support solutions and the medical.

9.5 Further Learning

The readers interested in learning more about medical image analysis and the role of image processing techniques in this manner are referred to [29–36].

Image processing and deep learning combinations are used in solving many different medical problems. As a very recent collection for understanding some about the current state, the readers can read [37–43].

As the world is currently (at the time of finalizing the book) dealing with the pandemic caused by the COVID-19 virus, there are also some recently published works focusing on image-based analyzes for coronavirus/COVID-19 diagnosis. Some of them are [44–49].

References

1. M. U. Akram, S. Khalid, S. A. Khan. Identification and classification of microaneurysms for early detection of diabetic retinopathy. Pattern Recognit. **46**(1): 107–116 (2013)
2. WHO. (2019). Blindness Causes. Online: http://www.who.int/blindness/causes/priority. Retrieved 28 Dec 2019
3. G. Quellec et al. Deep image mining for diabetic retinopathy screening. Med. Image Anal. 39: 178–193 (2017)
4. U. M. Akram et al. Detection and classification of retinal lesions for grading of diabetic retinopathy. Comput. Biol. Med. 45 (2014): 161–171. F. Chollet. (2015) Keras. Available: https://keras.io. Last accessed 2019/11/30
5. M. R. Mookiah, Krishnan et al. Computer-aided diagnosis of diabetic retinopathy: A review. Comput. Biol. Med. **43**(12): 2136–2155
6. K.S. Sreejini, V.K. Govindan, Severity grading of DME from retina images: A combination of PSO and FCM with bayes classifier. Int. J. Comput. Applications. **81**(16), 11–17 (2013)
7. L. Seoud, J. Chelbi, F. Cheriet, *Automatic Grading of Diabetic Retinopathy on a Public Database*, ed. by X. Chen, M. K. Garvin, J. J. Liu, E. Trusso, Y. Xu. Proceedings of the Ophthalmic Medical Image Analysis Second International Workshop, OMIA 2015, Held in Conjunction with MICCAI. (Munich, Germany, October 9, 2015), pp. 97–104. Available from https://doi.org/10.17077/omia.1032
8. U. R. Acharya, E. Y. K. Ng, J. H. Tan, An integrated index for the ident. J. Med. Syst. **36**(3): 2011–2020. https://doi.org/10.1007/s10916-011-9663-8
9. D. W. Safitri, D. Juniati, *Classification of Diabetic Retinopathy Using Fractal Dimension Analysis of Eye Fundus Image*. International Conference on Mathematics: Pure, Applied and Computation. AIP Conf. Proc. 1867, 020011-1–020011-11; https://doi.org/10.1063/1.4994414. (2017)
10. S.P. Savarkar, N. Kalkar, S.L. Tade, Diabetic retinopathy using image processing detection, classification and analysis. Int. J. Adv. Comput. Res. **3**(11), 585–588 (2013)
11. M.U. Akrametal, S. Khalid, S.A. Khan, Identification and classification of microaneurysms for early detection of diabetic retinopathy. Pattern Recogn. **46**, 107–116 (2013)
12. P. Chandrayan, Deep learning: Autoencoders fundamentals and types, https://codeburst.io/deep-learning-types-and-autoencoders-a40ee6754663. Son erişim 25 Ocak 2018
13. O. Deperlıoğlu, U. Köse, *Diagnosis of Diabetic Retinopathy by Using Image Processing and Convolutional Neural Network*. 2018 2nd International Symposium on Multidisciplinary Studies and Innovative Technologies (ISMSIT), (IEEE, 2018)

14. D. J. Hemanth, O. Deperlioglu, U. Kose, An enhanced diabetic retinopathy detection and classification approach using deep convolutional neural network. Neural Comput. Appl. (2019) https://doi.org/10.1007/s00521-018-03974-0
15. H. Pratt et al. Convolutional neural networks for diabetic retinopathy. Procedia Comput. Sci. 90: 200–205 (2016)
16. Kaggle, Diabetic retinopathy database. Online: https://www.kaggle.com/c/diabetic-retino pathy-detection/data. Retrieved 12 Feb 2020
17. J. Cuadros, G. Bresnick, EyePACS: An adaptable telemedicine system for dia- betic retinopathy screening. J. Diabetes Sci. Technol. 3(3), 509–516 (2009)
18. C. P. Wilkinson, F. L. Ferris, R. E. Klein, P. P. Lee, C. D. Agardh, M. Davis, D. Dills, A. Kampik, R. Pararajasegaram, J. T. Verdaguer, Proposed international clinical diabetic retinopathy and diabetic macular edema disease severity scales. Ophthalmology 110(9): 1677–1682 (2003). https://doi.org/10.1016/s0161-6420(03)00475-5
19. G. Quellec et al., Deep Image Min. Diabet. Retin. Screen. Med. Image Anal. 39, 178–193 (2017)
20. K. He, J. Sun, X. Tang, Single image haze removal using dark channel prior. IEEE Trans. Pattern Anal. Mach. Intell. 33(12), 2341–2353 (2010)
21. K. He, J. Sun, X. Tang, *Guided image filtering* (European Conference on Computer Vision, Springer, Berlin, Heidelberg, 2010)
22. S. Sabour, N. Frosst, G. E. Hinton, Dynamic routing between capsules. In *Advances in neural information processing systems*, (2017), pp. 3856–3866
23. A. Mobiny, H. Van Nguyen, *Fast Capsnet for Lung Cancer Screening.* International Conference on Medical Image Computing and Computer-Assisted Intervention, (Springer, Cham, 2018), pp. 741–749
24. H. Chao, L. Dong, Y. Liu, B. Lu, Emotion recognition from multiband EEG signals using CapsNet. Sensors 19(9), 2212 (2019)
25. W. Zhang, P. Tang, L. Zhao, Remote sensing image scene classification using CNN-CapsNet. Remote. Sens. 11(5), 494 (2019)
26. W. Zhang, J. Han, S. Deng, Heart sound classification based on scaled spectrogram and tensor decomposition. Biomed. Signal Process. Control 32, 20–28 (2017)
27. O. Deperlioglu, Classification of phonocardiograms with convolutional neural networks, brain. Broad Res. Artif. Intell. Neurosci. 9(2), 22–33 (2018)
28. D.J. Hemanth, O. Deperlioglu, U. Kose, An enhanced diabetic retinopathy detection and classification approach using deep convolutional neural network. Neural Comput. Appl. (2019). https://doi.org/10.1007/s00521-018-03974-0
29. J.S. Duncan, N. Ayache, Medical image analysis: Progress over two decades and the challenges ahead. IEEE Trans. Pattern Anal. Mach. Intell. 22(1), 85–106 (2000)
30. A. P. Dhawan, *Medical Image Analysis*, vol. 31, (Wiley, 2011)
31. A. Criminisi, J. Shotton, (eds.), *Decision Forests for Computer Vision and Medical Image Analysis*, (Springer Science & Business Media)
32. M. J. McAuliffe, F. M. Lalonde, D. McGarry, W. Gandler, K. Csaky, B. L. Trus, *Medical Image Processing, Analysis and Visualization in Clinical Research.* Proceedings 14th IEEE Symposium on Computer-Based Medical Systems (CBMS), (IEEE, 2001), pp. 381–386
33. J. L. Semmlow, B. Griffel, *Biosignal and Medical Image Processing*, (CRC press, 2014)
34. K. M. Martensen, *Radiographic Image Analysis-E-Book*, (Elsevier Health Sciences, 2013)
35. R. M. Rangayyan, *Biomedical Image Analysis.* (CRC press, 2004)
36. I. Bankman (ed.), *Handbook of Medical Image Processing and Analysis*, (Elsevier, 2008)
37. J.R. Hagerty, R.J. Stanley, H.A. Almubarak, N. Lama, R. Kasmi, P. Guo, W.V. Stoecker, Deep learning and handcrafted method fusion: Higher diagnostic accuracy for melanoma dermoscopy images. IEEE J. Biomed. Health Inform. 23(4), 1385–1391 (2019)
38. Y. Gurovich, Y. Hanani, O. Bar, G. Nadav, N. Fleischer, D. Gelbman, L.M. Bird, Identifying facial phenotypes of genetic disorders using deep learning. Nat. Med. 25(1), 60–64 (2019)
39. K. K. Wong, G. Fortino, D. Abbott, Deep learning-based cardiovascular image diagnosis: A promising challenge. *Future Generation Computer Systems*, (2019)

40. S. Dabeer, M.M. Khan, S. Islam, Cancer diagnosis in histopathological image: CNN based approach. Inform. Med. Unlocked **16**, 100231 (2019)
41. T. Jo, K. Nho, A.J. Saykin, Deep learning in Alzheimer's disease: Diagnostic classification and prognostic prediction using neuroimaging data. Front. Aging Neurosci. **11**, 220 (2019)
42. J. Xu, K. Xue, K. Zhang, Current status and future trends of clinical diagnoses via image-based deep learning. Theranostics **9**(25), 7556 (2019)
43. C.M. Dourado Jr., S.P.P. da Silva, R.V.M. da Nóbrega, A.C.D.S. Barros, P.P. Reboucas Filho, V.H.C. de Albuquerque, Deep learning IoT system for online stroke detection in skull computed tomography images. Comput. Netw. **152**, 25–39 (2019)
44. X. Xu, X. Jiang, C. Ma, P. Du, X. Li, S. Lv, L. Yu, Y. Chen, J. Su, G. Lang, Y. Li, *Deep Learning System to Screen Coronavirus Disease 2019 Pneumonia*. arXiv preprint arXiv:2002.09334. (2020)
45. I. D. Apostolopoulos, T. Bessiana, *Covid-19: Automatic Detection from X-ray Images Utilizing Transfer Learning with Convolutional Neural Networks*. arXiv preprint arXiv:2003.11617. (2020)
46. A. Narin, C. Kaya, Z. Pamuk, *Automatic Detection of Coronavirus Disease (COVID-19) Using X-ray Images and Deep Convolutional Neural Networks*. arXiv preprint arXiv:2003.10849. (2020)
47. S. Wang, B. Kang, J. Ma, X. Zeng, M. Xiao, J. Guo, M. Cai, J. Yang, Y. Li, X. Meng, B. Xu, *A Deep Learning Algorithm Using CT Images to Screen for Corona Virus Disease (COVID-19)*. medRxiv. (2020)
48. F. Shan, Y. Gao, J. Wang, W. Shi, N. Shi, M. Han, Z. Xue, Y. Shi, *Lung Infection Quantification of COVID-19 in CT Images with Deep Learning*. arXiv preprint arXiv:2003.04655. (2020)
49. L. Wang, A. Wong, *COVID-Net: A Tailored Deep Convolutional Neural Network Design for Detection of COVID-19 CASES From Chest Radiography Images*. arXiv preprint arXiv:2003.09871. (2020)

Chapter 10
Future of Medical Decision Support Systems

After having an introduction to the essential topics, the previous chapters have all provided effective use of deep learning for diagnosis of important diseases, as they are base for the medical decision support systems. There are of course many more research aspects to be discussed but if is also a good approach to focus on some insights regarding future of medical decision support systems.

Currently, there are many alternative technologies and innovative developments as bringing revolutionary changes for the humankind. As still the top place is kept by the field of artificial intelligence and its current sub-areas i.e. deep learning, future ideas can be better derived by thinking about possible topics that will greatly affect the future in terms of technological changes—developments, and making the modern life more practical and understandable. A very wide scope can be got if all factors shaping the future are thought but Fig. 10.1 represents a scheme of some of the foremost technologies as well as topics that can be considered as the components for the future scenarios of medical decision support systems.

As we should still think about the artificial intelligence, and deep learning, it is still unclear that the future may have new concepts. However, the role of intelligent systems will be still alive as they will be appearing common components in the context of different technologies and tools—devices. Based on the scope of the medical and relations to medical decision support systems, this chapter provides a final discussion for future developments in the following paragraphs.

10.1 Internet of Health Things and Wearable Technologies

Inter of Things (IoT) is known as a recent technology including intelligent communications of daily-life devices in the context of a network where data share, analyze and acting in a collaboration are all occurred accordingly [1–4]. Because of intense use of the digital world, it has been started to be influencing every task we do during

© The Editor(s) (if applicable) and The Author(s), under exclusive license to Springer Nature Singapore Pte Ltd. 2021
U. Kose et al., *Deep Learning for Medical Decision Support Systems*,
Studies in Computational Intelligence 909,
https://doi.org/10.1007/978-981-15-6325-6_10

Fig. 10.1 Some of the foremost technologies as well as topics that can be considered as the components for the future scenarios

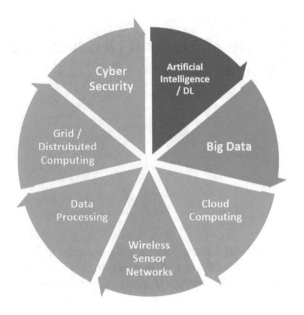

day. As computer as well as communication technologies such as Internet, wireless communication ensure critical roles in storing the information in the context of a digital world, the technological developments caused the IoT to rise as a great solution for an autonomous future with smart devices surrounding us to make everything easier and more practical (Of course there are many issues appearing within use of every technology, but that discussion regarding the IoT is another point of interest, as out of scope of this chapter/book). Briefly, IoT allows communicating among all devices that can take part in a network so data regarding people, environment, the other devices can be used accordingly for getting decision makings and performing some actions such as solving a tasks, adjusting the environmental factors, analyzing something or at least ensuring interaction with the people in order to inform them about the world around them. Here, advantages of IoT systems are indicated in Fig. 10.2.

All the mentioned advantages and the communication-oriented mechanisms of IoT are all because of innovative developments in artificial intelligence and the communication solutions such as wireless sensors, wireless communication standards, and also mobile technologies and communication approaches [5–8]. Nowadays, it is remarkable that IoT have already been widely used in different areas [9–13]. As that technology is more employed within a specific field, it is also re-called with new names, which are appropriate to the scope of the related field. Internet of Health Things (IoHT) is among them.

IoHT is briefly a type of IoT that is applied for medical applications [14, 15]. Because the future will be probably with full of autonomous devices, use of IoT as well as IoHT will be probably a common thing because the field of medical will be always at the first places to benefit from innovative technologies. In accordance to

Fig. 10.2 Advantages of
Internet of Things systems

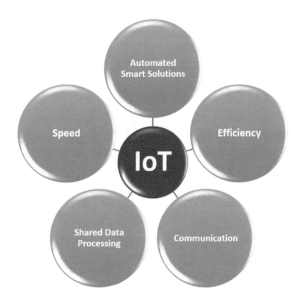

that, the future of medical decision support systems will include intense use of IoHT systems. In detail, possible scenarios will be like as follows:

- After getting up in the morning smart mirrors and cameras in our houses will support us to be ready to the day and they will also track for any mood changes or possible illness.
- Toilets will be devices analyzing urine and stool to make diagnosis of diseases and/or early diagnosis of experiencing bad-way life standards.
- All our medical data will be kept in secure over blockchain running encrypted cloud so that all smart devices will be decision making about our health state.
- Our cars will be tracking our health state and possible tiredness symptoms.
- While working at office environment, smart devices will be tracking our performance as well as mental and health state against any disease or lowering in our well-being.
- Surgeries will be made by decision-making smart robotic systems accurately and in a faster manner.
- All treatments will be tracked by smart devices around us so that we will be faster recovering.
- Thanks to early actions by smart devices, people will not easily be infected or at least be preventing themselves from possible diseases.
- Smart devices will support us to have healthy food and track our medical data for a healthy aging in time.

Since it is still possible to imagine more and more about the possible future scenarios, IoHT here ensure a critical role for supporting us for having good health and well-being generally. As IoHT systems of the future will be associated with deep learning (any maybe more advanced forms with new names), the analyzing,

Fig. 10.3 Essential benefits to be provided by the future IoHT systems

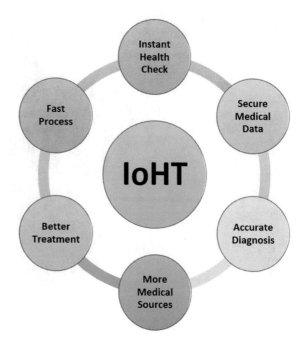

diagnosing, and treatment processes will be even faster and more effective according to today. Covering all the explanations so far, Fig. 10.3 provides essential benefits to be provided by the future IoHT systems.

As associated with the IoHT perspective, the future of medical decision support systems will be also with wearable technologies. Currently, there are many different types of wearable technologies ready to be used (Fig. 10.4 [14]). Wearable technologies can effectively track our data and ensure smart features to support us for an easier life and even decision making generally. Considering the medical, wearable technologies will be probably common components of IoHT upper-systems and will be essential tools for understanding more about us and people for ensuring general well-being.

10.2   Robotics

When a discussion on artificial intelligence and the future is made, the robotics technologies are certain topic that is widely explained. As appropriate to that, the future of the medical decision support systems will be intensively associated with more use of robotics. Even nowadays, there are many examples of robotics usage in different fields and it is already a constant component of the future [16–18]. In the context of medical problems and decision support tasks, the following scenarios can be thought accordingly:

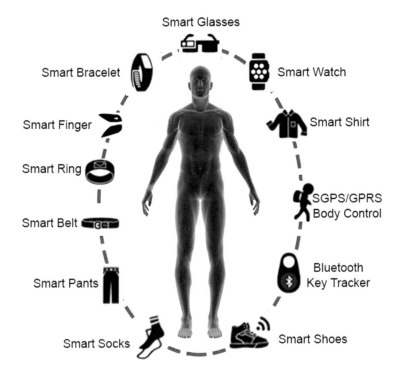

Fig. 10.4 Wearable technologies today [14]

- In the future, there will be kiosk-like robotic systems serving public spaces for helping people for simple medical diagnosis and treatments.
- As surgeries are already supported by hard and soft robotics [19, 20], the future will be including wider use of robotics during surgery. Such robotic systems will not only be performing—supporting the surgery but will also help doctors in decision making processes.
- Artificial intelligence is already used in physical rehabilitation applications [21–23]. In the future, there will be more rehabilitation robots and at homes, people (especially older people) will be supported by personal assistant robots with medical knowledge.
- Many of simple medical tests (i.e. taking blood sample) at hospitals will be made by service robotics.
- There will be advanced diagnosis robotics-based rooms for performing general check-up processes.
- Medical tasks that are generally dangerous to be done by humans will be done by robots.
- There will be more use of soft robotics because of their advantages according to hard robotics.

- There will be more robotic expert systems performing answer-question related interactions with people, in order to get ideas about health state, possible disorders/diseases, and collection pre-information for supporting doctors in decision making.
- Robotic systems will be probably even in smaller and as integrated to wearable technologies for better tracking purposes.

10.3 Information and Drug Discovery

As it was mentioned and emphasized in the previous chapters, information discovery is among critical solution ways of the artificial intelligence. Thanks to deep learning and big data use, information discovery has gained more momentum in time. Information discovery can be used to derive new combination of information, wider knowledge and new patterns resulting to the exact mechanism-role of the discovery [24, 25].

Diseases has always been problem for the humankind. Currently, the humankind is even experiencing a pandemic caused by the coronavirus COVID-19 and because of that almost all research works of medical has directed to finding effective treatment of COVID-19. That situation and past experiences with different diseases, which were strong then and weak (or eliminated) nowadays indicate the importance of using information discovery for the drug discovery done with the employment of artificial intelligence in the field of medical. Moving from that, the future will intensively include running drug discovery (discovering medicine—vaccine as well as treatment strategies) by employing effective algorithms—techniques and running them in the context of advanced decision support systems. For even nowadays, there are many examples of drug discovery studies done with deep learning [26–31] so that future diseases, viral infections, disorders and new type of micro-organisms will be often subject to drug discovery studies. Here drug discovery can be an effective step of a whole medical health management system, including use of intelligent systems for analyzes, diagnosis, drug discovery and then treatment processes in the context of a decision support flow, as illustrated in Fig. 10.5.

10.4 Rare Disease and Cancer Diagnosis

Use of automated medical diagnosis as the component of medical decision support systems has already been a good weapon of the humankind for all kinds of diseases. As indicated under the previous paragraph, the future of medical will be still including dealing with infections, micro-organisms and maybe today's vital disease: cancer will be still analyzed, diagnosed and then treated with the use of intelligent systems running medical support systems. Currently, there are already research works done

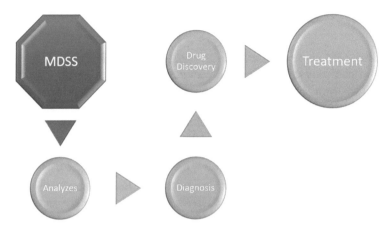

Fig. 10.5 Decision support flow with different steps to be done by intelligent systems

for effective diagnosis of different cancer types [32–42]. With especially good collaboration with image processing, deep learning architectures have been effectively using against cancer diagnosis (Fig. 10.6). On the other hand, there is also rare diseases including i.e. viral, bacterial infections (when they are not pandemic yet), specific allergies, and genetical disorders [43–45]. As some of technological tools and changes in life standards are also affecting directly or indirectly human metabolism and causing rare diseases, there will be still need for medical decision support systems to deal with rare diseases, too. Since it is also possible to ensure a balanced, healthy life thanks to i.e. IoHT systems as explained before, there is still possibility of rare diseases or cancers as there is the chaos in the universe and the nature. However, future intelligent systems will be key factor to deal with such issues, as a remarkable insight for the future.

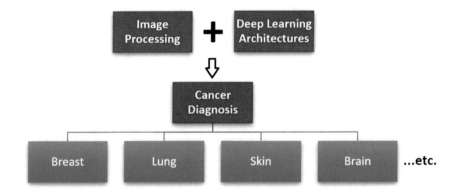

Fig. 10.6 Image processing and deep learning use against cancer diagnosis

10.5 COVID-19 and Pandemics Control

As indicated before, the humankind is currently (at the time of writing that section of this chapter; March 2020) dealing with the coronavirus type: COVID-19 and it became a pandemic in a short time. Because of the COVID-19, governments around the world has applied remarkable policies including breaks at works, schools, universities with remote—online working conditions at homes, quarantines for preventing people from getting COVID-19, which causes deaths in remarkably short times. As general, there is a great emergency state, which is something like the life around the world stopped. That situation has shown researchers to effective use of technology for early diagnosis of such viral infections before they become pandemics or at least running effective treatments and discoveries (i.e. vaccine) rapidly for eliminating that devastating disease. Nowadays, there are already research works focusing on use of artificial intelligence/deep learning for diagnosis of COVID-19 and deriving alternative treatments for it [46–56]. Since that problem has taught many things to the humankind, it can be clearly expressed that the future of medical decision support systems will include pandemics control approaches with deeper analyze and tracking of the data around the world. At this point, a possible system scenario can be expressed briefly as follows (Fig. 10.7):

- The key point in the system is using as much as remote communication possibilities in order to keep near contact of humans against any viral infection appearance. In order to ensure that the IoHT system will be common components of the COVID-19 and pandemic control system.

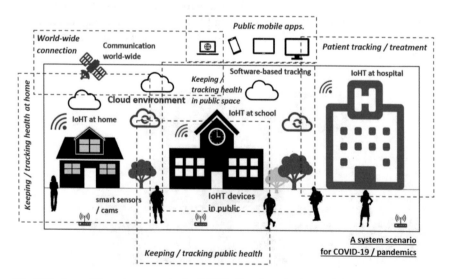

Fig. 10.7 A possible system scenario for COVID-19 and pandemics control

- IoHT based devices will be connected world-wide over cloud systems and the data security will be ensured with effective technologies such as blockchain [57, 58] or tangle [59, 60]. World-wide communication of IoHT based devices will be organized with efficient, optimized approaches and models based on globally accepted standards.
- IoHT devices will include especially following groups of devices: (1) patient tracking and treatment devices at hospitals, (2) public health support devices spread around cities, roads, restaurants, schools, and similar public places, (3) personal health tracking devices at homes (these may be revised according to needs). Roles of these devices will include especially followings:

  - (1) Patient tracking and treatment devices will be used at hospitals for as far as possible interaction with the patients and tracking states of the patients with viral—bacterial diseases remotely. That will also allow doctors, medical staff to track everything in even remote mode and using i.e. e-signatures to give orders or perform any tasks that can be done remotely. Eventually, near interactions of people will be as low as possible except from cases such as surgeries, emergency actions—diagnosis.
  - (2) Public health support devices will support people to keep themselves clean and in safe against diseases. Also, these devices will give people advices, announce emergency states, and ensuring trainings for keeping awareness at a desired level. These devices will also in contact with cleaning services and any other sustainability—green environment technologies in the context of IoT/IoHT.
  - (3) Personal health tracking devices will be responsible to check all people's health state in the same home environment and direct them or ensure communication with hospitals/doctors remotely in case of any suggestions, regular checks, or emergency state predictions.

- As the whole three groups of devices will be in connect with each other, it will be possible to control a virus infection case, by i.e. keeping infected people at home and acting to treat them in accordance to the quarantine rules, perform remote checks—controls at hospitals, improving level of tasks to be done by IoHT devices in public spaces, and many more tasks to do collaboratively by IoHT devices running over artificial intelligence, sensor technologies, mobile communication channels, secure algorithms, and additional technologies to achieve a global, accurate smart system.
- Public spaces will be supported with intense use of sensors, cameras, and drones for achieving better IoT-oriented communication as well as tracking actions for people—public health.
- There will be world-wide software environment allowing public tracking of world-wide viral infections, and also detailed tracking for authorized users such as doctors, policy makers, governments, as having changing authorization levels.
- There will be world-wide up-to-date agreements such as medical data regarding viral—bacterial diseases/infections will be shared instantly around the globe, by securing patient personal data, and the countries will be responsible to share their

data of such diseases/infections with an upper-commission or i.e. World Health Organization.

- There will be of course specially designed diagnosis, treatment technologies and separate smart hospitals, quarantine houses—hotels in case of any pandemic.
- There will be artificial intelligence/deep learning based accurate—fast diagnosis systems, intelligent vaccine development kits, and may be robotics-based services for remote treatment of patients with virus. Analyzes, predictions, control of smart—intelligent systems will be all supported with Data Science and artificial intelligence solutions.
- Thanks to the synergy ensured among IoHT devices world-wide, it will be possible for every people to track spreading of any pandemic instantly, like it is an online streaming video or instantly changing data such as economic time series. As that can be done with mobile applications, such applications will also ensure effective communications, announcements world-wide and country-specific.
- *All the explained working mechanism of the scenario may be revised—updated with addition of alternative technologies, and more use of detailed tasks in control of pandemics such as COVID-19.*

As it can be understood, use of intelligent systems as well as data control—tracking solutions (use of Data Science generally) will give important advantages to the humankind for fighting against pandemics like COVID-19. It is clear that the more a medical decision support system is structured over combinations of solution techniques, the more it could be robust and sustainable for vital medical tasks like predicting, tracking, controlling, treating pandemics.

10.6 Summary

The future of medical decision support systems is all wide open for further research and innovative developments. As a result of improvements and rapid developments in different technologies, the outcomes have always been effective on practical technological solutions for daily-life. After the twenty-first century, that state has been experiencing widely in all different fields. As a critical field, medical will always keep its top place for the newest solutions. Here, solutions by intelligent systems will be key triggering factor for both solving medical problems as well as taking it steps away for better well-being of the humankind.

As also a final touch to this book, this chapter discussed some specific subjects, which the authors think will be important for the future of medical decision support systems. The explanations including IoT, IoHT, wearable technologies, robotics, drug discovery, diagnosis of cancers as well as rare diseases are important topics for further research. Of course, as the current threat for the existence of the humankind, COVID-19 and pandemics have been also discussed in the sense of their control and treatment, as the final, vital topic.

As concluding comments for the book, the authors have provided a current view on use of deep learning for rising medical decision support systems. Employment of different deep learning architectures, using them for especially diagnosis solutions so forming essentials of medical decision support systems are rapidly improving research topics so that there will be always need for such reference book for better understanding the latest research and having future ideas. The authors would like to thank all readers for reading that book and desire to see same interests for the future works by them.

10.7 Further Learning

In order to have some more future insights from very recent works regarding future of artificial intelligence as well as its role in medical, readers can read [61–76].

For learning more about smart medical applications (with especially support by IoT, mobile communication, and some other technologies) as well as some future perspectives, the readers are referred to [77–81].

References

1. L. Tan, N. Wang, Future internet: the internet of things, in *2010 3rd International Conference on Advanced Computer Theory and Engineering (ICACTE)*, vol. 5. (IEEE, 2010), pp. V5–376)
2. L. Atzori, A. Iera, G. Morabito, The internet of things: a survey. Comput. Netw. **54**(15), 2787–2805 (2010)
3. A. McEwen, H. Cassimally, *Designing the Internet of Things* (Wiley, 2013)
4. S.C. Mukhopadhyay, N.K. Suryadevara, Internet of things: challenges and opportunities, in *Internet of Things.* (Springer, Cham, 2014), pp. 1–17
5. P. Waher, *Learning Internet of Things* (Packt Publishing Ltd., 2015)
6. L. Da Xu, W. He, S. Li, Internet of things in industries: a survey. IEEE Trans. Ind. Inf. **10**(4), 2233–2243 (2014)
7. Z. Abbas, W. Yoon, A survey on energy conserving mechanisms for the internet of things: wireless networking aspects. Sensors **15**(10), 24818–24847 (2015)
8. E. Ahmed, I. Yaqoob, A. Gani, M. Imran, M. Guizani, Internet-of-things-based smart environments: state of the art, taxonomy, and open research challenges. IEEE Wirel. Commun. **23**(5), 10–16 (2016)
9. N. Shahid, S. Aneja, Internet of things: vision, application areas and research challenges, in *2017 International Conference on I-SMAC (IoT in Social, Mobile, Analytics and Cloud)(I-SMAC)* (IEEE, 2017), pp. 583–587
10. N. Dlodlo, J. Kalezhi, The internet of things in agriculture for sustainable rural development, in *2015 International Conference on Emerging Trends in Networks and Computer Communications (ETNCC).* (IEEE, 2015), pp. 13–18.
11. P. Pruet, C.S. Ang, D. Farzin, N. Chaiwut, Exploring the internet of "educational things" (IoET) in rural underprivileged areas, in *2015 12th International Conference on Electrical Engineering/Electronics, Computer, Telecommunications and Information Technology (ECTI-CON)* (IEEE, 2015), pp. 1–5

12. N. Papakostas, J. O'Connor, G. Byrne, Internet of things technologies in manufacturing: application areas, challenges and outlook, in *2016 International Conference on Information Society (i-Society)*. (IEEE, 2016), pp. 126–131

13. R. Ramakrishnan, L. Gaur, Smart electricity distribution in residential areas: Internet of Things (IoT) based advanced metering infrastructure and cloud analytics. In *2016 International Conference on Internet of Things and Applications (IOTA)* (IEEE, 2016), pp. 46–51

14. J.J. Rodrigues, D.B.D.R. Segundo, H.A. Junqueira, M.H. Sabino, R.M. Prince, J. Al-Muhtadi, V.H.C. De Albuquerque, Enabling technologies for the internet of health things. IEEE Access **6**, 13129–13141 (2018)

15. E. Tsekleves, R. Cooper, Design research opportunities in the internet of health things: a review of reviews (2018)

16. B. Siciliano, & O. Khatib (eds.), *Springer Handbook of Robotics* (Springer, 2016)

17. T.R. Kurfess (ed.) *Robotics and Automation Handbook* (CRC Press, 2018)

18. S. Madakam, R.M. Holmukhe, D.K. Jaiswal, The future digital work force: robotic process automation (RPA). JISTEM-J. Inf. Syst. Technol. Manage. **16** (2019)

19. T.L. Ghezzi, O.C. Corleta, 30 years of robotic surgery. World J. Surg. **40**(10), 2550–2557 (2016)

20. J. Guo, J.H. Low, X. Liang, J.S. Lee, Y.R. Wong, R.C.H. Yeow, A hybrid soft robotic surgical gripper system for delicate nerve manipulation in digital nerve repair surgery. IEEE/ASME Trans. Mechatron. **24**(4), 1440–1451 (2019)

21. M. Papakostas, V. Kanal, M. Abujelala, K. Tsiakas, F. Makedon, Physical fatigue detection through EMG wearables and subjective user reports: a machine learning approach towards adaptive rehabilitation, in *Proceedings of the 12th ACM International Conference on PErvasive Technologies Related to Assistive Environments* (2019), pp. 475–481

22. D. Novak, R. Riener, Control strategies and artificial intelligence in rehabilitation robotics. Ai Mag. **36**(4), 23–33 (2015)

23. M.H. Lee, D.P. Siewiorek, A. Smailagic, A. Bernardino, S. Bermúdez i Badia, Interactive hybrid approach to combine machine and human intelligence for personalized rehabilitation assessment, in *Proceedings of the ACM Conference on Health, Inference, and Learning* (2020), pp. 160–169

24. A. Moukas, Amalthaea information discovery and filtering using a multiagent evolving ecosystem. Appl. Artif. Intell. **11**(5), 437–457 (1997)

25. M. Steyvers, P. Smyth, M. Rosen-Zvi, T. Griffiths, Probabilistic author-topic models for information discovery, in *Proceedings of the Tenth ACM SIGKDD International Conference on Knowledge Discovery and Data Mining* (2004), pp. 306–315

26. L. Zhang, J. Tan, D. Han, H. Zhu, From machine learning to deep learning: progress in machine intelligence for rational drug discovery. Drug Discovery Today **22**(11), 1680–1685 (2017)

27. A. Korotcov, V. Tkachenko, D.P. Russo, S. Ekins, Comparison of deep learning with multiple machine learning methods and metrics using diverse drug discovery data sets. Mol. Pharm. **14**(12), 4462–4475 (2017)

28. Y. Jing, Y. Bian, Z. Hu, L. Wang, X.Q.S. Xie, Deep learning for drug design: an artificial intelligence paradigm for drug discovery in the big data era. AAPS J. **20**(3), 58 (2018)

29. B. Ramsundar, P. Eastman, P. Walters, V. Pande, *Deep Learning for the Life Sciences: Applying Deep Learning to Genomics, Microscopy, Drug Discovery, and More*. (O'Reilly Media, Inc., 2019)

30. B.J. Neves, R.C. Braga, V.M. Alves, M.N. Lima, G.C. Cassiano, E.N. Muratov, F.T. Costa, C.H. Andrade, Deep learning-driven research for drug discovery: tackling malaria. PLoS Comput. Biol. **16**(2), e1007025 (2020)

31. H. Zhu, Big data and artificial intelligence modeling for drug discovery. Annu. Rev. Pharmacol. Toxicol. **60**, 573–589 (2020)

32. R. Fakoor, F. Ladhak, A. Nazi, M. Huber, Using deep learning to enhance cancer diagnosis and classification, in *Proceedings of the International Conference on Machine Learning*, vol. 28 (ACM, New York, USA, 2013)

33. W. Sun, B. Zheng, W. Qian, Computer aided lung cancer diagnosis with deep learning algorithms, in *Medical Imaging 2016: Computer-Aided Diagnosis*, vol. 9785. (International Society for Optics and Photonics, 2016), p. 97850Z

34. S. Liu, H, Zheng, Y. Feng, W. Li, Prostate cancer diagnosis using deep learning with 3D multiparametric MRI, in *Medical Imaging 2017: Computer-Aided Diagnosis*, vol. 10134 (International Society for Optics and Photonics, 2017), p. 1013428

35. W. Sun, T.L.B. Tseng, J. Zhang, W. Qian, Enhancing deep convolutional neural network scheme for breast cancer diagnosis with unlabeled data. Comput. Med. Imaging Graph. **57**, 4–9 (2017)

36. Z. Han, B. Wei, Y. Zheng, Y. Yin, K. Li, S. Li, Breast cancer multi-classification from histopathological images with structured deep learning model. Sci. Rep. **7**(1), 1–10 (2017)

37. Y. Zeng, S. Xu, W.C. Chapman Jr., S. Li, Z. Alipour, H. Abdelal, D. Chatterjee, Q. Zhu, Real-time colorectal cancer diagnosis using PR-OCT with deep learning. Theranostics **10**(6), 2587 (2020)

38. N. Zhang, Y.X. Cai, Y.Y. Wang, Y.T. Tian, X.L. Wang, B. Badami, Skin cancer diagnosis based on optimized convolutional neural network. Artif. Intell. Med. **102**, 101756 (2020)

39. S. Alheejawi, M. Mandal, H. Xu, C. Lu, R. Berendt, N. Jha, Deep learning-based histopathological image analysis for automated detection and staging of melanoma, in *Deep Learning Techniques for Biomedical and Health Informatics* (Academic Press, 2020), pp. 237–265

40. J.H. Lee, E.J. Ha, D. Kim, Y.J. Jung, S. Heo, Y.H. Jang, S.H. An, K. Lee, Application of deep learning to the diagnosis of cervical lymph node metastasis from thyroid cancer with CT: external validation and clinical utility for resident training. Eur. Radiol. 1–7 (2020)

41. W. Bulten, H. Pinckaers, H. van Boven, R. Vink, T. de Bel, B. van Ginneken, J. van der Laak, C. Hulsbergen-van de Kaa, G. Litjens. Automated deep-learning system for Gleason grading of prostate cancer using biopsies: a diagnostic study. Lancet Oncol. (2020)

42. Y.Q. Jiang, J.H. Xiong, H.Y. Li, X.H. Yang, W.T. Yu, M. Gao, X. Zhao, H. Gu, Using smartphone and deep learning technology to help diagnose skin cancer. Br. J. Dermatol. **182**(3), e95–e95 (2020)

43. M. I. Qadir, (ed.) *Rare and Uncommon Diseases* (Cambridge Scholars Publishing, 2018)

44. T.F. Boat, M.J. Field (eds.), *Rare Diseases and Orphan Products: Accelerating Research and Development* (National Academies Press, 2011)

45. S.C. Groft, M.P. de la Paz, Preparing for the future of rare diseases, in *Rare Diseases Epidemiology: Update and Overview* (Springer, Cham, 2017), pp. 641–648

46. L. Huang, R. Han, T. Ai, P. Yu, H. Kang, Q. Tao, L. Xia, Serial quantitative chest CT assessment of COVID-19: deep-learning approach. Radiol.: Cardiothor. Imaging **2**(2), e200075 (2020)

47. I.D. Apostolopoulos, T. Bessiana, Covid-19: automatic detection from X-Ray images utilizing transfer learning with convolutional neural networks (2020). arXiv:2003.11617

48. F. Shan , Y. Gao , J. Wang, W. Shi, N. Shi, M. Han, Z. Xue, Y. Shi, Lung Infection quantification of COVID-19 in CT images with deep learning (2020). arXiv:2003.04655

49. L. Li, L. Qin, Z. Xu, Y. Yin, X. Wang, B. Kong, J. Bai, Y. Lu, Z. Fang, Q. Song, K. Cao, Artificial intelligence distinguishes COVID-19 from community acquired pneumonia on chest CT. Radiology 200905 (2020)

50. S. Wang, B. Kang, J. Ma, X. Zeng, M. Xiao, J. Guo, M. Cai, J. Yang, Y. Li, X. Meng, B. Xu, A deep learning algorithm using CT images to screen for Corona Virus Disease (COVID-19) (2020)

51. L. Wang, A. Wong, COVID-Net: a tailored deep convolutional neural network design for detection of COVID-19 cases from chest radiography images (2020). arXiv:2003.09871

52. C.J. Huang, Y.H. Chen, Y. Ma, P.H. Kuo, Multiple-input deep convolutional neural network model for COVID-19 forecasting in China (2020)

53. X. Xu, X. Jiang, C. Ma, P. Du, X. Li, S. Lv, L. Yu, Y. Chen, J. Su, G. Lang, Deep learning system to screen coronavirus disease 2019 pneumonia (2020). arXiv:2002.09334

54. A. Narin, C. Kaya, Z. Pamuk, Automatic detection of coronavirus disease (COVID-19) using X-ray images and deep convolutional neural networks. (2020). arXiv:2003.10849

55. E. Ong, M.U. Wong, A. Huffman, Y. He, COVID-19 coronavirus vaccine design using reverse vaccinology and machine learning (2020)

56. A. Zhavoronkov, V. Aladinskiy, A. Zhebrak, B. Zagribelnyy, V. Terentiev, D.S. Bezrukov, D. Polykovskiy, Y. Yan, Potential COVID-2019 3C-like protease inhibitors designed using generative deep learning approaches. Insilico Med. Hong Kong Ltd. A **307**, E1 (2020)

57. D. Drescher, *Blockchain Basics*, vol. 276 (Apress, Berkeley, CA, 2017)

58. Z. Zheng, S. Xie, H.N. Dai, X. Chen, H. Wang, Blockchain challenges and opportunities: a survey. Int. J. Web Grid Serv. **14**(4), 352–375 (2018)

59. T. Alsboui, Y. Qin, R. Hill, Enabling distributed intelligence in the internet of things using the IOTA tangle architecture, in *4th International Conference on Internet of Things, Big Data and Security* (SciTePress, 2019), pp. 392–398

60. M. Divya, N.B. Biradar, IOTA-next generation block chain. Int. J. Eng. Comput. Sci. **7**(04), 23823–23826 (2018)

61. A. Alexander, A. Jiang, C. Ferreira, D. Zurkiya, An intelligent future for medical imaging: a market outlook on artificial intelligence for medical imaging. J. Am. Coll. Radiol. **17**(1), 165–170 (2020)

62. A.C. SolbergK.E. Müller, C.T. Solberg, Artificial intelligence and the future art of medicine. Tidsskrift for Den norske legeforening (2020)

63. V. Jahrreiss, J. Veser, C. Seitz, M. Özsoy, Artificial intelligence: the future of urinary stone management? Curr. Opin. Urol. **30**(2), 196–199 (2020)

64. L. Floridi, What the near future of artificial intelligence could be, in *The 2019 Yearbook of the Digital Ethics Lab* (Springer, Cham, 2020), pp. 127–142

65. G. Briganti, O. Le Moine, Artificial Intelligence in medicine: today and tomorrow. Front. Med. **7**, 27 (2020)

66. H. Rivas, Future entrepreneurship in digital health, in *Digital Health Entrepreneurship* (Springer, Cham, 2020), pp. 215–219

67. K.K. Sharma, S.D. Pawar, B. Bali, Proactive preventive and evidence-based artificial intelligene models: future healthcare, in *International Conference on Intelligent Computing and Smart Communication 2019* (Springer, Singapore, 2020), pp. 463–472

68. M. Bhandari, T. Zeffiro, M. Reddiboina, Artificial intelligence and robotic surgery: current perspective and future directions. Curr. Opin. Urol. **30**(1), 48–54 (2020)

69. E.B. Sloane, R.J. Silva, Artificial intelligence in medical devices and clinical decision support systems, in *Clinical Engineering Handbook* (Academic Press, 2020), pp. 556–568

70. Y.W. Chen, K. Stanley, W. Att, Artificial intelligence in dentistry: current applications and future perspectives. Quintessence Int. **51**, 248–257 (2020)

71. O.F. El-Gayar, L.S. Ambati, N. Nawar, Wearables, artificial intelligence, and the future of healthcare, in *AI and Big Data's Potential for Disruptive Innovation* (IGI Global, 2020), pp. 104–129

72. A. Chang, The role of artificial intelligence in digital health, in *Digital Health Entrepreneurship* (Springer, Cham, 2020), pp. 71–81

73. P.M. Doraiswamy, C. Blease, K. Bodner, Artificial intelligence and the future of psychiatry: insights from a global physician survey. Artif. Intell. Med. **102**, 101753 (2020)

74. C. Webster, & S. Ivanov, Robotics, artificial intelligence, and the evolving nature of work, in *Digital Transformation in Business and Society* (Palgrave Macmillan, Cham, 2020), pp. 127–143

75. K.S. Mudgal, , N. Das, The ethical adoption of artificial intelligence in radiology. BJR Open **2**(1), 20190020 (2020)

76. S. Dalton-Brown, The ethics of medical ai and the physician-patient relationship. Camb. Q. Healthcare Ethics **29**(1), 115–121 (2020)

77. A. Ahad, M. Tahir, K.L.A. Yau, 5G-based smart healthcare network: architecture, taxonomy, challenges and future research directions. IEEE Access **7**, 100747–100762 (2019)

78. S. Tuli, N. Basumatary, S.S. Gill, M. Kahani, R.C. Arya, G.S. Wander, R. Buyya, Healthfog: an ensemble deep learning based smart healthcare system for automatic diagnosis of heart diseases in integrated IoT and fog computing environments. Future Gener. Comput. Syst. **104**, 187–200 (2020)

79. A. Ghani, Healthcare electronics—A step closer to future smart cities. ICT Express **5**(4), 256–260 (2019)
80. G. Sannino, G. De Pietro, L. Verde, Healthcare systems: an overview of the most important aspects of current and future m-health applications, in *Connected Health in Smart Cities* (Springer, Cham 2020), pp. 213–231
81. O. F. El-Gayar, L.S. Ambati, N. Nawar, Wearables, artificial intelligence, and the future of healthcare, in *AI and Big Data's Potential for Disruptive Innovation* (IGI Global, 2020), pp. 104–129

Printed in the United States
by Baker & Taylor Publisher Services